Hoping to Help

A volume in the series

THE CULTURE AND POLITICS OF HEALTH CARE WORK

Edited by Suzanne Gordon and Sioban Nelson

For a list of books in the series, visit our website
at www.cornellpress.cornell.edu.

Hoping to Help

The Promises and Pitfalls of Global Health Volunteering

Judith N. Lasker

ILR Press

AN IMPRINT OF

Cornell University Press

Ithaca and London

For Shira and Ariella
and
For the students who have inspired
and collaborated with me in this work

They will surely continue to make the
world better by their presence in it

First published 2016 by Cornell University Press
First printing, Cornell Paperbacks, 2016

Printed in the United States of America

Library of Congress Cataloging-in-Publication Data

Lasker, Judith, 1947– author.
  Hoping to help : the promises and pitfalls of global health volunteering
/ Judith N. Lasker.
    pages cm. — (The culture and politics of health care work)
  Includes bibliographical references and index.
  ISBN 978-1-5017-0009-5 (cloth : alk. paper) —
  ISBN 978-1-5017-0010-1 (pbk. : alk. paper)
  1. Volunteer workers in medical care. 2. Missions, Medical.
3. Medical assistance—International cooperation. 4. Voluntary health
agencies. I. Title.
  RA972.7.L37 2016
  362.1—dc23   2015029553

Cornell University Press strives to use environmentally responsible
suppliers and materials to the fullest extent possible in the publishing of
its books. Such materials include vegetable-based, low-VOC inks and
acid-free papers that are recycled, totally chlorine-free, or partly composed
of nonwood fibers. For further information, visit our website at
www.cornellpress.cornell.edu.

Cloth printing   10 9 8 7 6 5 4 3 2 1
Paperback printing   10 9 8 7 6 5 4 3 2 1

printed with union labor

Contents

Acknowledgments

Authors know that they are indebted to the ideas, labor, patience, and assistance of others, and that is certainly the case for this book. Many colleagues, students, friends, and family members have helped me along on this exciting journey. I have tried to remember them all, and I apologize for any omissions.

First, my students and research assistants who have contributed ideas, data analysis, bibliographic research, and more: Julien Armstrong, Kave Bulambo, Nikki Daddaria, Mari Freedberg, Tamara Huson, Joshua Lynn, Anna Patterson, Leah Paulson, Allison Prosswimmer, Nicholas Rockwell, Lauren Rothenberg, Christina Simone, Nishika Vidanage, Alessandra Bazo Vienrich, and Adrienne Viola.

Four students in particular contributed to this project by participating in short-term volunteer trips and carrying out research before and after: Sirry Alang, who traveled to Ghana with the first Becton Dickinson (BD) trip I was involved with as her research adviser; Caroline Kusi, who went on a subsequent BD trip to Ghana and then returned there with me for follow-up research; Ana Arteaga, who accompanied me to Haiti on a trip organized by Heart to Heart International and sponsored by BD and who helped in carrying out interviews there; and Joe Rendon, who traveled with me to Ecuador on a trip sponsored by Timmy Global Health and who acted as translator as well as interviewer.

The invitation by Becton Dickinson leadership and staff to involve Lehigh students as well as me in their Volunteer Service Trips led directly to this book, and I will forever be grateful for their generosity and assistance. Thanks go in particular to Matt Mattern, Eugene Vivino, Jennifer Farrington, Paula Kapotes, and Kathy Zimmerman. The collaboration of Heart to Heart International was indispensable in making the research in Haiti possible. Thanks so much especially to Steve Hower, Amy Beil, Josh Jakobitz, and Carla Orner. Matt MacGregor generously invited me to join a Timmy Global Health Brigade in Ecuador, and the staff there, including August Longino and Valerie Matron, was very welcoming and helpful.

Thank you especially to the dozens of Haitian and Ecuadorian staff members whom I met and interviewed and who were so welcoming to my students and me. Thanks as well to the hospital staff members in Kumasi, Ghana, interviewed by Caroline Kusi, and to Susan Rosenfeld and the staff she interviewed in Niamey, Niger. Susan also transcribed and translated her interviews. Karen Myers provided outstanding service as a transcriptionist for the many English language interviews.

Thanks as well to the scores of others who participated in this research, either by responding to my survey or by participating in interviews. The book is greatly enriched by the insights and experiences of all the participants, those who sponsor volunteer trips, those who volunteer, those who welcome the volunteers in host countries, and the global health experts I interviewed.

Research requires not only dedicated and capable associates and participants but also funding. Lehigh University support has made it possible for me to travel and hire research assistants and to have the time to carry out the research. My NEH professorship fund and a Faculty Incentive Grant were especially helpful for this project. Thank you to Anne Meltzer and Alan Snyder for providing time and funding and to Lehigh staff members who assisted me with administrative and budget issues—Erica Nastasi, Nancy Dwyer, and Laura Chiles.

The Brocher Foundation in Geneva was an ideal place to spend three months working on the initial draft of this manuscript. Thanks to Dena Davis for encouraging me to apply and helping with the details, and to the staff at Brocher for providing housing, food, office space, and colleagues and for making my stay there so enjoyable and productive.

I was fortunate to be asked by Bruce Compton, Global Health Director at Catholic Health Association, to work on a study of short-term medical mission trips that involved staff at Catholic hospitals and health systems in the United States. He and Father Michael Rozier, S.J., were excellent collaborators in that project and made it possible for me to include valuable data that added to this book.

I am grateful to friends and colleagues who encouraged me along the way with valuable suggestions, information, and reading of parts of the manuscript. These include in particular Kelly Austin, Seth Goren, Gail Gulliksen, Eric Hartman, Allan Kellehear, Ben Lough, Ziad Munson, Ruth Nathanson, Myra Rosenhaus, Ruth Setton, Stephanie Short, Ariella Siegel, Shira Siegel, Ellen Sogolow, Kevin Sykes, David Walker, and Bruce Whitehouse.

A very special thanks to Scott Cooper for his skillful and thoughtful editing. Fran Benson and Suzanne Gordon of Cornell University Press offered valuable feedback on the manuscript. Thanks also to Dave Prout for the index.

My fabulous daughters, Shira Siegel and Ariella Siegel, were always my greatest cheerleaders, and I cannot begin to express adequately how much their love and support has meant to me.

I am grateful to all these people, named and unnamed, and to others who have written about and studied short-term volunteering.

INTRODUCTION

A "Tsunami" of Volunteers

The developing world has become a playground for the redemption of
privileged souls looking to atone for global injustices.

—Ossob Mohamud, Somalian blogger, *Guardian* online, February 2013

"Voluntourists" they may be—but their work can have a huge impact on
their own lives and the lives of those they help.

—Sam Blackledge, British newspaper reporter, *Guardian* online,
February 2013

Medical missions. Health brigades. Flying surgeons. Hundreds of thousands of people from the wealthier countries of the world travel annually to poorer countries for brief service trips as volunteers in programs sponsored by a growing number of community churches and national religious organizations, nonprofits large and small, colleges and schools of medicine and public health, hospitals, major corporations, and tourist agencies promoting "volunteer vacations." Nearly every time I mention my research, someone has a personal experience to recount or tells me about a family member or close friend who has volunteered. That was not the case only a decade ago.

The number of people involved in volunteer activities is staggering. An estimate done between 1995 and 2000 concluded that the number of domestic and international volunteers contributing through voluntary organizations in thirty-six countries, when taken together, would com-prise the world's ninth-largest country in terms of population.[1] Those numbers have increased significantly in the years since.

Focusing on international volunteer activities originating in the United States alone, Lough and colleagues used census data to conclude in 2007 that about 1 million Americans volunteer in other countries each year. They estimated that these volunteers spend 162 million hours on international volunteering, valued (based on the hourly rate assigned to volunteer work by the Independent Sector) at close to $3 billion; today, using the same method, that figure is $3.6 billion.[2] Twenty-one percent of people whose volunteering is *primarily* international reported providing counseling or medical care,[3] so the annual number of American global health volunteers is at least two hundred thousand, and the value is currently more than $750 million.

This number estimates the value of volunteer time, but there are many hundreds of millions more in direct costs involved, which have not been counted. The majority of the money spent on international volunteering never gets to the countries that host volunteers. About half goes to airlines, and much of the rest pays for the cost of administration and supplies pro-vided in the United States.[4]

In February 2013, the *Guardian* newspaper in London published, on its online Guardian African Network site, what turned out to be a debate over what has been called "voluntourism." The Somalian blogger Ossob Mohamud, in a contribution titled "Beware the 'voluntourists' doing good," wrote, "Voluntourism almost always involves a group of idealistic and privileged travelers who have vastly different socio-economic statuses vis-à-vis those they serve. They often enter these communities with little or no understanding of the locals' history, culture, and ways of life. All that is understood is the poverty and the presumed neediness of the com-munity, and for the purposes of volunteering that seems to be enough. The developing world has become a playground for the redemption of privi-leged souls looking to atone for global injustices by escaping the vacuity of modernity and globalisation."[5]

Mohamud's piece generated a lot of reaction, including a response from Sam Blackledge, a senior reporter on the *Plymouth* (England) *Herald* staff. "No approach is without its flaws," he wrote, "but it is vital that people do not group charities doing this well with companies who are putting very little into the developing world. Charities that invest in the developing world need keen, energetic, ambitious people to help them along. 'Voluntourists' they may be—but their work can have a huge impact on their own lives and the lives of those they help. It would be an awful shame if they were put off."[6]

The exchange between Mohamud and Blackledge encapsulates the division between those who believe international volunteering is beneficial, indeed essential, and those who argue that it has too many problems and causes more harm than good.

How do we know who is right? What evidence exists to support these conflicting views? Although short-term international volunteering is a massive and growing enterprise, there is very little information about what volunteers do, where they go, who is sponsoring them, and what they accomplish. Assessing the value of this enterprise must start with a much better understanding of what it looks like, from the perspective of both sponsors and host communities.

There isn't even a common definition of "short-term." When I began this research, I thought trips of six months or less should be included. Therefore, when I contacted organizers, I asked them about volunteer trips of this duration. Yet I learned from conducting two national surveys of organizers in the United States that the vast majority of volunteer trips last two weeks or less.[7]

In this book I focus on these brief health-related volunteer programs. The programs include both primary care and more advanced hospital and surgical interventions; prevention, such as improving water and sewage systems; health education; and medical training. As we will see, interest in "global health" in the United States and other countries is growing very rapidly and generating a huge demand for opportunities to help and learn in this domain. Yet many of the recommendations could be applied to other kinds of international volunteering—for example, those that focus on educational or environmental programs.

Short-term volunteering can have many benefits for the organizations that sponsor programs, the companies from which they purchase goods and services, and the individual volunteers who may gain in personal growth, credentials for careers, and bragging rights. But what are the benefits, and the costs, for host communities? Can these efforts be designed in such a way as to maximize the benefits (as in Blackledge's reference to "charities doing this well") and minimize potential harm? It is a challenge—but one worth undertaking.

Dr. Edward O'Neil, founder and president of Omni Med, one of the thousands of organizations that send volunteers to poor countries to provide medical care and health education, aptly identifies the need for better assessment.

> When those with long-term experience in developing countries speak of programs that send international volunteers, they often do so with skepticism or disdain—and not without reason. The field of global volunteerism is littered with the wreckage of the well-intentioned but poorly informed. While some service programs are models of efficiency, efficacy, and intelligent construction, . . . others base their program designs on what seems right, with little to no evidence for proceeding and even less monitoring and evaluation. Those of us who live and work in this space know that many programs have made and continue to make an enormous difference in the world. However, there is simply no data to back up this claim.[8]

So many of the people who spend time and money to volunteer in other countries do so because, as they will tell you, they are "giving back." These volunteers acknowledge the good fortune in their own lives, and they feel a sense of obligation to help others. These motives are to be applauded. But we must still ask whether these mostly well-meaning efforts actually improve people's lives.

Some volunteer programs enhance, and sometimes even save, lives. Others have very little effect on the host communities. Still others may cause harm. The best programs incorporate key qualities identified in this book and referred to later as "Principles for Maximizing the Benefits of Volunteer Health Trips." I have come to these principles after extensive interviews with host-country staff, organizers, and volunteers; surveys of sponsoring organizations; and participant observation, as well as input from the work of others. Some of them may seem obvious, but they are all too often ignored.

I have learned that a major portion of programs do very cursory screening of volunteers and barely prepare them for the country they will be visiting and the work they will be doing. Too many have no local partners to work with in determining the local needs and the best ways to address them. Too many organizations arrive in countries only sporadically (as described by one program director, a group might show up in a village unexpectedly and ring the bell for patients to come), with no continuity of programming and no follow-up to services offered to address possible complications. Most do not send volunteers for a long enough period to benefit the hosts or the volunteers optimally. And almost none evaluate the impact of their presence on host communities.

The best programs promote mutuality between hosts and visitors and continuity of programming. The best programs also collaborate with communities to carry out a needs assessment and involve the local staff at every step. Ideally, they focus on prevention and on integration of services. Longer stays are better than shorter ones, and language and cultural preparation makes a difference. Capacity building matters. Evaluating programs, and then incorporating the results into program improvements, is crucial—but it is rare.

It is too simple to paint the entire volunteer phenomenon with a single brush, either all glowing and shiny or all dismal and ugly. It is also insufficient to ask, as some people do, whether the benefits are greater for volunteers or for hosts; this is not a two-sided phenomenon but actually one with three main sets of actors, each of which is analyzed in its own section of the book. As we will see later, many benefits accrue to sponsoring organizations in the wealthy countries from sending volunteers on short-term medical trips. The question, "Who benefits?" must take their interests into account.

My hope is that this book will contribute valuable information and perspectives to the widening debate about short-term volunteering so that organizers, funders, volunteers, and hosts—all those who are "hoping to help"—can aim for the best use of precious resources in helping to make the lives of people throughout the world as healthy as possible.

Here Come the Volunteers

On a weekend in June 2012, I stood at the airport in Port-au-Prince, Haiti, and watched while groups of North Americans rotated in and out of the country for one-week volunteering projects at orphanages, building sites, health clinics, and

churches throughout the island nation. A group from New Brunswick, Can-
ada, had come to build houses designed to be earthquake resistant; they would
use rubble from the devastating 2010 earthquake as material. Another group
from State College, Pennsylvania, was in Haiti to do construction work on an
orphanage. College students and their pastor/adviser from Georgia Baptists for
Haiti—wearing T-shirts emblazoned with "Preach, Teach, Heal, Build"—
spent a week working in an outpatient clinic. Other groups of people I saw at
the airport were also wearing matching T-shirts identifying their organizations
and emblazoned with slogans such as "Hope for Haiti."

The large numbers of arrivals and departures at the airport reminded me
in some ways of the weekly Saturday turnover at American time-share vaca-
tion resorts. Hundreds check out; hundreds more check in. But here they were
coming in groups, with purpose and with the idea that they would make a
difference.

Volunteers and the organizations that send them for short periods to
poorer countries often describe the trips as "missions" or "brigades." Both
words describe organized, purposeful ventures to accomplish a goal. "Mission" has been used in religious contexts; "brigade" is primarily a military
term. In whatever use, both words denote a group with a purpose, a calling, and a common cause.[9]

What I am exploring here is the *purpose* of these missions and brigades
and whether these hundreds of weekly arrivals really bring hope (or housing or health benefits) to Haiti or to the thousands of other poor communities around the world that receive international volunteers every year. It
may seem obvious that the goal is to accomplish good for the communities visited, to "make a difference," and often to "give back." Whether this
actually happens, and what other objectives might be involved in these
volunteer trips, is rarely considered. These issues motivate this book. Do
volunteers help or hurt? In what ways? Can these missions be handled
more effectively?

My interest in this topic intensified a few years ago when I began working with students who went on short-term health-related volunteer service trips sponsored by a major corporation. My students accompanied
employees and worked on research projects, reporting their findings to
corporate leadership after each trip. The three students who participated
in these excellent opportunities returned with many questions and with

suggestions about how the volunteer project could have been improved for all concerned.

Each of these three students was born outside the United States—two in Africa and one in Latin America. Perhaps their concerns were sharpened by their backgrounds, which gave them a different perspective from that of many volunteers from wealthy countries. But I have also had many American-born students who have participated in volunteer trips and returned wondering aloud whether they had made any difference.

These students all asked the same questions I'm asking here, even if in different ways. They had departed with great enthusiasm and returned excited about and grateful for their experiences. But in some cases they were deeply troubled about whether their trips had led to improved health for the residents of the countries visited or whether they had mainly served the interests of the volunteers and their organizations.

The conventional wisdom in the "sending" countries is that health-related volunteering *must* be a good thing for the host-community members because it has to be better than having no volunteers at all.[10] After all, they bring medicine and skills and equipment to areas lacking them, and that must be beneficial.

When I ask whether the enormous expenditure of money and time represented by short-term volunteering produces the best possible result for the health of residents of the countries visited, some insist it's the wrong question. They see the benefits more in terms of the impact on volunteers, who are presumed to gain greater intercultural and international understanding and may be influenced to work for greater justice in their future. One man who heard me speak about my research commented somewhat angrily. "I want my son to learn to be charitable," he exclaimed, "and this is a way to do that. So why are you even questioning its value?"

As a social scientist, my response is to expand my questions to ask whether this is the best way for a young person from a wealthy country to "learn to be charitable." I wonder what this son and his peers can learn from a week or two in a poor country. *Do* they become more charitable? *Do* they become advocates for justice or more culturally aware? Some observers believe they do, while others worry that volunteers may come away with distorted impressions that actually perpetuate some of the very problems they hope to alleviate.[11] And again, the evidence is mostly lacking.

Many people believe volunteers help improve the health of people in poor countries, but others are convinced they do not. Indeed, many people consider it a self-serving, colonialist-like adventure with as great a potential for harm as for good. Of course, the reality is much more complex than a simple determination that volunteering is good or bad, and I have endeavored to present a more nuanced account based on research carried out both in the United States with sponsoring organizations and in four host countries with teams who work with volunteers.

Fortunately, many people who sponsor volunteer programs *do* want to know whether their involvement actually has an impact. Organizers and prospective participants alike are interested in gaining a better understanding of whether what they are doing makes a difference for the people they hope to help. The enormous human and economic investment in volunteer trips should prompt a desire in everyone involved to know more about how these precious resources are invested and whether this is the best way to improve the lives of people in poor communities of the world. Everyone involved must focus on how to make this effort as valuable as possible.

And what an effort it is. The explosive increase in international health volunteering in the past two decades—Dr. Neal Nathanson vividly compares it to a tsunami—is driven by several forces. Nathanson, founding associate dean for Global Health Programs at the University of Pennsylvania Medical School, asked students how they would explain the increased interest: "They don't know. 9/11? CNN? Rwanda? . . . They want to help; it's something visceral, a tidal wave sweeping the country, a tsunami, something in the air. They are responding to their visceral impulse. 'There is so much need, and I want to be part of the solution.' Not any further than that."

There are, of course, many forces that contribute to the form in which these desires and opportunities are expressed.

What Drives the Growth of International Volunteering?

Volunteering is much more than an individual decision to offer service to others. Often it is the product of purposeful policymaking with the goal of serving a variety of priorities at many different levels, including international, national, and corporate. And while there have been medical

missionaries and international volunteers for centuries, we are now looking at a fairly recent and complex phenomenon that has been actively fos-
tered by many powerful actors for a large variety of reasons.

The world's poorest countries have seen a sharp decline in public services. Privatization of health services resulted in part from Structural
Adjustment Programs required by the World Bank and International
Monetary Fund in response to mounting foreign debt crises in the early
1980s.[12] These policies, emerging from a growing dominance of neoliberal ideology favoring the private sector, have led in many places to
a severe decline in basic services formerly offered, however poorly, by
national governments. At the same time, the HIV/AIDS pandemic created overwhelming new demands for services and a tremendous and
tragic loss of educated and skilled personnel in many countries. The recent Ebola epidemic in West Africa and civil wars and refugee crises in
many parts of the world vastly exacerbate this situation in the countries
affected.

Claire Wendland, a physician and anthropologist from the University
of Wisconsin who spent two decades providing medical care and doing
anthropology field work in Malawi, highlights the increasing degradation
of basic public services she observed: "Public hospitals and clinics have
visibly deteriorated under the triple pressures of budget austerity measures, increasing population, and a huge surge in HIV-related illnesses.
Nearly every medication and supply—including such basics as sutures and
iodine—ran out on a regular basis during the years of my fieldwork there.
Staffing was so skeletal that one clinical officer might care for several hundred inpatients in a district hospital, and one nurse might be responsible
for a ward of 60."[13]

These are the kinds of conditions that spur outside organizations to set
up alternative hospitals and clinics staffed by volunteers. Awareness of the
needs also drives major fundraising campaigns in wealthy countries to
support programs that intend to address the needs.

The decline in public services described by Wendland has been accompanied by changes in the types of needs. In past years, the major health
issue in poor countries was infectious diseases, many of which were addressed by large-scale vaccination, sanitation, and education campaigns.
With the partial or complete success of some international campaigns and
subsequent increase in life expectancy, noncommunicable diseases such as

diabetes and hypertension are becoming more prominent in the health and mortality profile of countries everywhere in the world. Poor countries have experienced a sharp increase in chronic ailments that require ongoing and regular medical attention, yet this type of service is too often unavailable in many parts of the world. At the same time, infectious diseases continue to kill many people prematurely. This has been referred to as the "double burden" of disease in poor countries.[14]

All of this unfolds within the context of increased globalization and changing geopolitics since the mid-1990s. Arturo Escobar describes a new "geopolitical formation" that resulted in "securitization of development," the end of the "Washington consensus" (widely accepted views about development that dominated the practices of powerful institutions since the 1970s), and the disappearance of socialism as an alternative.[15]

These changes have motivated many individuals and organizations in the wealthier countries to take on some of the goals of development not met by previous efforts or models and thus contributed to the rise of volunteering. Jim Butcher and Peter Smith, who have been studying volunteer tourism, agree that these fundamental political and ideological changes have driven the increase in volunteering, an activity they refer to as an example of "life politics," which focuses on individual identity rather than grand political narratives for acting on one's environment. They note that the growth of life politics in contemporary life represents a move away from "collective solutions to social problems towards individual life choices." This shift occurred, they argue, as a result of the collapse of Communism and the end of the Cold War, leading to a "far-reaching 'crisis of meaning' . . . that pushes ethical consumption to the fore." With no clear societal model offering an alternative to the market economy, individualistic approaches received a boost, and individual volunteering as a strategy for change was one of the results.[16]

The same forces are likely contributing to the enhanced involvement of private corporations in international volunteering. Some have described the increased role of corporations in social services "as part of the rolling back of the state across the world"[17]—not unlike the explanation for the increase in nongovernmental organizations (NGOs). Notably, companies often frame as "investment" what used to be considered "gifts"—another shift that can be linked to the dominance of neoliberal ideology regarding the primacy of the market.

Mass media help fuel the increase in volunteering by publicizing need in poorer countries. Celebrities, too, draw attention through their advocacy work, going back to the highly publicized events such as Band Aid's Christmas recording in 1984, the Live Aid concert in 1985, and many examples since.[18] In more recent years, there has been a great deal of attention to Sean Penn's post-earthquake efforts in Haiti, volunteer work done by the British princes in Chile and Malawi, and Oprah Winfrey's creation of a school for girls in South Africa. CNN began an annual "Heroes" contest in 2006 to bring attention to individuals who have begun innovative programs in response to specific problems such as sex trafficking and hunger.[19] All of these create dramatic, well-publicized examples that others may want to imitate.

The Internet and social media, too, have played a big role. They make it much easier to find out about volunteer opportunities and share experiences with others. Indeed, organizations responding to my survey listed the Internet as the main method of recruitment for organizations seeking volunteers.

"Communication is there at markedly increased rates of speed through social media," Dr. Mark Rosenberg, CEO of the Task Force for Global Health, told me. "YouTube alone would be enough to account for this, but that's just one facet of people's increasing awareness of what's going on, that we live on the whole planet and that the United States is not totally isolated and insulated from the rest of the world. I also think there's increasing awareness of the disparities in terms of health status and access to good health and access to the means of health. I think increasingly people see that it's not very equitable."

As individual awareness of volunteering opportunities has grown, many national governments are now providing considerable encouragement and financial support for volunteering.[20] It is maddening that the reductions in the social safety nets of poorer countries promoted by many of these same governments and by international financial institutions such as the World Bank and International Monetary Fund have created the very need to which those same actors have responded by promoting volunteer interventions.

In some cases, the goal of governments in supporting volunteering is to provide an alternative to military service; in others, it is to foster a positive image of the country among people in other nations or to build civic engagement as a practice among citizens.[21]

In the United States, it has become customary for presidents to promote volunteering. President George H. W. Bush had his "Thousand Points of Light." In 1993, President Clinton created AmeriCorps (including domestic and international service organizations), the size of which President George W. Bush increased in 2002. In 2009, President Obama signed into law the Edward M. Kennedy Serve America Act, which called for a further increase in positions in the AmeriCorps program from 75,000 to 250,000 by 2017 and the creation of four national service corps.[22]

Similar trends are seen in Europe. Two thousand six saw the launching of the Manifesto for Volunteering in Europe by a network of thirty-eight volunteer development agencies and centers. The manifesto states that "voluntary action is . . . an important component of the strategic objective of the European Union of becoming the most competitive and dynamic, knowledge-based economy in the world."[23]

At an even broader level, the United Nations created the United Nations Volunteers (UNV) division in 1997 and declared 2001 to be the International Year of the Volunteer, an event celebrated in 130 countries[24] and followed by conferences and reports in succeeding years. In 2011, UNV released "State of the World's Volunteerism Report; Universal Values for Global Well-being," with a focus "on the universal values that motivate people the world over to volunteer for the common good and on the impact of volunteer action on societies and individuals."[25] The United Nations itself sponsors eight thousand volunteers annually; the majority of them are from developing countries.[26]

Most of the explanations for increased international volunteer activity focus on meeting unmet needs. But we cannot lose sight of the motives for gain, a number of which are explored in this book. Nations pursuing political and security goals, individuals seeking personal advantages, and companies seeking profits also contribute to the growth of this phenomenon.

The tourism industry is one example of the latter; agencies have discovered that potential customers can more easily justify a major expenditure on travel if it is tied to an altruistic venture and is not just for pleasure. Many cruise lines offer one-day service opportunities as excursions in the countries they visit.[27]

Increased wealth makes volunteering possible for the more privileged residents of countries in the global North, who must pay their own expenses or find donors to assist, whether through their churches, their schools, their employers, or NGOs.[28] And the experience of volunteering may well enhance that privilege, as those who can afford to embark on international missions gain experience and credentials. Questions about justice and equality are necessarily part of any analysis of this growing enterprise.

All the activities that encourage volunteerism unfold in the context not only of a decline in public services but also against a backdrop of widespread criticism of foreign aid. In light of publicity about waste, inefficiency, and the harmful consequences of many such programs, as well as concerns about the many unmet needs at home, it is perhaps not surprising that the majority of the American public believes that the U.S. government spends more on foreign aid than it should (and more than it actually does).[29] But we must seriously ask whether volunteers, sponsored mostly by private organizations and enabled by private donations and their own ability to pay their expenses, can do better.

The Critiques

As short-term international volunteer programs become ever more popular, they have also been the target of criticism. Among the epithets: "drive-by humanitarianism,"[30] "fistula tourism,"[31] and "slum tourism."[32] Nigerian American writer Teju Cole posted a series of comments to Twitter about the "white savior industrial complex," which he called the "fastest growth industry in the US."[33] The growing involvement of privileged people in programs in poor countries has even been referred to as a new form of colonialism, a comparison I will return to in the final chapter.[34]

The criticisms also take the form of very specific concerns about whether short-term medical missions are helpful or harmful to host communities.[35] For instance, Daniel A. Guttentag, a professor at the University of Waterloo in Canada, writes that most studies of what he calls "volunteer tourism" are overwhelmingly positive about its value, but that these studies focus almost entirely on the value for volunteers. As a response, he lists what he considers five possible negative impacts.[36]

First, there is "a neglect of locals' desires." To make recruitment effective, a program may be more focused on the volunteer's satisfaction than on host needs. The quality of those volunteers leads to the second on the list: "A hindering of work progress and the completion of unsatisfactory work." Volunteers are often unskilled, and they may need attention that interrupts an organization's work, or they may do poor-quality work.

When volunteers work on construction projects that could be done by local residents, they may be undercutting employment opportunities in the host community. This leads to Guttentag's third negative impact: "A decrease in employment opportunities and a promotion of dependency." Volunteerism can also promote deference to outside expertise, diminishing self-sufficiency.

The fourth and fifth impacts on Guttentag's list are considerably broader. One is "reinforcement of conceptualisations of the 'other' and rationalizations of poverty." Many volunteers do not change their own attitudes but may reinforce a dualistic conception of us-them, the latter defined by simplistic images of poverty. Or they may rationalize poverty by focusing on impressions of "poor but happy" people. Further, volunteers' belongings and wealth may affect local values and consumption patterns, which Guttentag calls "instigation of cultural changes, caused by the demonstration effect."

Ian Birrell, a British journalist who has written extensively about the popular volunteer option of visiting orphanages in poor countries, captures many of the criticisms that are also made of medical missions. In a 2010 column in the *Guardian* (London), he describes some of the negative impacts.

> Wealthy tourists prevent local workers from getting much-needed jobs, especially when they pay to volunteer; hard-pressed institutions waste time looking after them and money upgrading facilities; and abused or abandoned children form emotional attachments to the visitors, who increase their trauma by disappearing back home. . . . In Africa, tour firms throw in a visit to an orphanage alongside a few days on the beach or watching wild animals. Critics argue that dropping in to take photographs of orphaned children, who may have seen parents recently waste to death, reduces them to the status of lions and zebras on the veld. Many orphanages let tourists work with children. But what would we say if unchecked foreigners went into our children's homes to cuddle and care for the kids?

We would be shocked, so why should standards be lowered in the developing world?[37]

This may seem harsh, but each aspect of Birrell's critique has been mentioned by people writing about medical missions: the competition with local workers, both health professionals and the unskilled; the voyeurism toward and objectification of poor people; and the free access to patients and children given to people without proper credentials or screening.

Such critiques can be disturbing in an era when there is growing demand, especially in wealthier countries, for international service opportunities; when the needs are great; and when overall the media have given admiring attention to humanitarian trips. The idea that groups of nineteen-year-olds with energy and good intentions and "Hope for Haiti" emblazoned on their T-shirts should be anything but applauded will strike many as surprising, even offensive. Even greater offense might be taken when surgeons who use their vacation time every year to travel to remote locations and operate on patients and train local physicians are subjected to criticism.

Despite the criticisms, dedicated (and sometimes just curious or adventurous) volunteers continue to flock to and spend their own money on programs designed to help fill the huge gaps in public health and medical services in poor countries. At issue is whether that energy and those financial and human resources are used to benefit poor communities to the maximum extent.

Most of the conflicting assessments of short-term volunteering reflect the views of people in the global North—the wealthier countries that send most volunteers. But it is crucial to know what people in the host communities—the global South—think. Their voices have rarely been heard in this debate, which is why I devote so much space in this book to recounting what they have to say. What do they see as the value of having volunteers come to their communities? What, in their opinions, are the qualities of the good volunteers, and what describes the ones who are not so welcome? What are the best kinds of volunteer programs in terms of benefit to their communities?

Of course, not all short-term volunteering is the same, but the criticisms must be taken seriously. The most frequently published critiques have appeared in medical journals and address the important ethical problem of allowing medical students to work far beyond their training in communities with few resources.[38] My concern here is primarily with a larger ethical question: whether the investment of billions of dollars of resources in the short-term volunteering enterprise can be justified by the results in terms of improvement in health, reduction in health disparities, or other measures of value to the host communities.

The director of a large volunteering organization, who has dedicated his career to creating short-term volunteer services, told me,

> If short-term occasional health services were the best way to get medical care, we'd be doing it in our own countries, and obviously we are not. We know that short-term trips are not the perfect way to provide healthcare services. But we also know that there is an incredible demand for healthcare services in poor areas, and an incredible supply of volunteers that want to support projects around the world. The trick, then, should be to improve the way in which these volunteers provide services, minimizing the negatives of short-term trips and maximizing the positives, while also supporting the capacity of local healthcare systems.

His comment is a poignant reminder of how far these programs are from creating ideal conditions for improving health but also of the challenge to volunteer program sponsors to make programs as beneficial as possible.

To begin to get a handle on how short-term volunteering can provide the most benefit for all people involved, we need to know more about the three major parties in this enterprise—the sponsoring organizations, the volunteers, and the host communities. We need to consider the size, scope, and widely varying characteristics of short-term health-related volunteering. That includes further understanding what motivates volunteers and organizations to undertake these trips. It involves looking at the characteristics of these service programs—what they do and where and how they partner with organizations in the host countries. It means exploring the goals of the different types of sponsoring organizations and how they might conflict with the needs of people in the host countries. And finally, it requires asking what qualities of programs and volunteers are most likely to be useful to both volunteers and host communities.

Ultimately, my goal is not to advocate for all volunteering or to call for its dismantling. Rather, I hope to contribute to making it more effective and valuable to all concerned.

A Note on Data and Study Participants

My research includes both quantitative data from a survey of U.S. sending organizations and qualitative findings from interviews and observations, both designed to gain an understanding of the nature of short-term health volunteering. This approach provides multiple viewpoints while allowing for cross-checking the validity of results from each type of method. (Further details on methodology, including an explanation of how I selected the organizations studied, are in Appendix A.)

My research associates and I interviewed 119 people, including 55 host-country staff members in four countries in Africa, Latin America, and the Caribbean; 15 volunteers; 27 officials of U.S. sponsor organizations; 15 American and French staffers working full-time in host countries who have worked with volunteers; and 7 global health experts.

I also conducted an Internet survey of U.S.-based organizations that send volunteers overseas for short-term health programs. Responses represent 177 different organizations. Each year these organizations send, in total, an estimated 20,637 volunteers to other countries for health projects. That averages out to 119 per organization. Some individual organizations send fewer than 10, while others send as many as 1,500 in one year. Educational institutions, on average, send fewer volunteers than other types of organizations (half of them send 25 or fewer), while NGOs report the highest number of volunteers, with more than one-third sending 100 or more volunteers per year.

I refer at times to results of a similar survey on which I collaborated, which was distributed by the Catholic Health Association to its member hospitals and health systems in the United States. We received responses from 152 organizers of short-term medical missions and 205 recent volunteers on such trips.

Additionally, my students (with me or under my supervision) observed medical missions, conducted pre- and post-surveys of volunteers and host-country trainees as well as focus groups with the latter, and made follow-up visits to mission hosts for interviews and focus groups.

All participants were assured they would not be named without their permission, and no host-country staff members are identified by name. Officials of sponsor organizations, global health experts, and expatriates working with volunteers are identified only if they approved the quotes attributed to them. Others are identified only by generic descriptions of their positions.

Part I

THE SPONSORING ORGANIZATIONS

Each year, thousands of organizations large and small send hundreds of thousands of volunteers to work in health-related projects in other countries. Volunteer programs vary a great deal in their history, the types of activities they engage in, and their models for programming, but certain patterns emerge as they are studied.

In order to understand the impact of international health volunteering, we need to know more about who is sponsoring these activities, what they hope to accomplish, where they go, and what they do. We will see that the volunteering enterprise reflects the goals and history that sponsoring organizations bring to it, as well as the larger social forces that have driven its growth.

1

Who Sponsors International Medical Missions?

Most of the volunteer programs I write about began in the last two decades, a time of tremendous growth in NGOs and in university-based international activities. Volunteer organizations, though, have been working in other countries for a long time. For example, Catholic Medical Mission Board dates its origin to 1912 and has worked in 123 countries. Project Hope launched its traveling hospital ship in 1958 and has taken it to 35 countries. Operation Smile was founded in 1982 to provide cleft palate repair and surgical training in poor countries; in recent years, it has expanded to offer dentistry and burn care. These and other organizations operate worldwide and raise millions of dollars each year.

Individual physicians have founded many international volunteer organizations. They are driven by a desire to make a difference and often also by religious faith. Their destination choices are most often a product of personal history or chance encounters rather than an analysis of where needs are greatest. The choice of focus—primary care, surgery, screening, or health education—is also a product of perceived need or of personal capabilities rather than any kind of systematic assessment.

Types of Organizations

The great majority of organizations that send volunteers from wealthy countries to poorer countries to work in health-related projects fall into one of four major types:[1]

- Faith-based organizations
- Nongovernmental organizations that are *not* faith based
- Educational organizations
- Corporate groups

Most are nonprofit entities. Some, particularly the NGOs, were created specifically to sponsor volunteer activities. Others have broader goals and activities, of which international volunteering is one part. For example, the volunteers who go on short-term health-related trips for educational institutions and corporations tend to come from the ranks of the students or employees of these organizations, and service trips are only a small part of the overall organizational mission. Since the 1990s, a growing number of for-profit commercial firms offer fee-paying "voluntary work" placements.[2] These broker firms may create their own service projects or just connect volunteers to existing projects. They often consult with universities or corporations to help them offer volunteer opportunities to students or employees.[3]

The responses to my national survey of volunteer organizations encompass three of these groups, with faith-based organizations dominating.[4] The small number of corporations that directly sponsor international health volunteering were not included in the survey. They are, however, an important and increasing presence, and I discuss them later.

To get a deeper sense for what these organizations are about and how they became engaged in the world of global health volunteering, we need to look more closely at their origins and growth. Most have stories that reveal how their different goals and personal experiences have helped define their programs and their choices about where to send volunteers.

"Pap Smears for Jesus"? Religious Volunteer Organizations

I am attending a 2013 conference on Christian medical missions with more than five hundred other people. We meet in a large nondenominational church in the

Midwest for a weekend of workshops, plenary sessions, and exhibits by many Christian organizations that are there to recruit volunteers or publicize their activities in sending supplies to poor countries. Some sessions are straight medical information—how to deliver emergency care in resource-poor settings, for example. Others focus on how to use medical care to serve an evangelical purpose.

The attendees gather for the opening session in the huge sanctuary. The first speaker is a convert to Christianity who tells us, "God is going to use you to serve someone, and that will raise up attention for a bigger conversation. Meet the need, but something bigger is going on. Meeting people's needs leads them to ask you why you're there."

Another speaker is a physician who asks us not to tell others her name or the place where she has been working, since missionary work is forbidden there. She tells us that God has given her the opportunity to use her gifts of medicine to work with people who have little access to medical care or to the Gospel.

Another medical missionary reports that she prays with 80 percent of patients, and they see that it works. She claims that her prayers healed a schizophrenic. Her advice to the audience: "Take the opportunity to tell people about Christ. Don't come home bragging about seeing five hundred patients if you didn't use the opportunity to talk about the Gospel. Be a servant. It's all about Jesus first, medicine second. Don't be a jerk. You're there to serve people. That is what Jesus did."

I begin with faith-based organizations because the origins of volunteering can be traced primarily to religion and because they comprise by far, the largest component of current short-term volunteering. Just over half of those who responded to my survey identified their organizations as "faith-based." As Dr. Mark Rosenberg, CEO of the Task Force for Global Health, told me, "The early history of global health was very much dominated by missionaries and mission groups trying to do good."

To this day, the largest numbers of American volunteers, whether they serve domestically or internationally, are connected to religious organizations.[5] The Princeton sociologist Robert Wuthnow estimates that 1.6 million church members travel on short-term international mission trips each year.[6] The anthropologists Robert Priest and Brian Howell estimate that "upwards of two million" North Americans per year go on short-term missions. These estimates are not all for health-related mission trips.[7]

And not all of them adopt the type of evangelism advocated by many speakers at the conference I attended. In fact, many deeply devout volunteers object to including any preaching in the services they provide. For example, one physician who regularly travels with a religious organization expressed strong disapproval of the purveyors of what she calls "Pap smears for Jesus." As we will see in this chapter, faith-based organizations that sponsor international trips in which volunteers offer health-related services (often referred to as "medical missions") adopt three quite different approaches to the role of faith in their activities.

The scope of faith-based volunteering is vast; from international missionary branches of major Christian denominations, many founded more than a century ago, to small groups organized by one or two leaders for specific projects, faith-based overseas volunteering groups cover the widest variety of programs.

Just about every major Christian denomination has a missionary branch operating in many parts of the world, with medical care often a central part of the work. The United Methodist Church's Volunteers in Mission project supports a "global health initiative." The Catholic Medical Mission Board's Medical Volunteer Program operates in many countries to provide clinical care and public health interventions. The Presbyterian Church (USA) has a mission branch with a program in International Health and Development. These are but a few examples. The list of churches and church-sponsored hospitals with international medical missions is long and includes Seventh-Day Adventists, Church of the Nazarene, the Episcopal Church, Mormons, and various Catholic orders such as the Salesians and Maryknoll. Hospitals and health systems founded by Catholic and other religious organizations sponsor many short-term medical missions overseas, as do a very large number of independent faith-based NGOs.

Then there are the thousands of volunteers from individual parishes doing work that is not coordinated through any denominational body or larger faith-based volunteering organization. Typically, these trips involve either onetime or occasional missions with local church members and are not usually advertised or affiliated with any national efforts. Most often the trips are carried out in partnership with specific churches in the host country and have a focus on Bible study and assisting the congregation with projects such as construction or repairs on the church building. But some also include bringing medical supplies and setting up onetime health clinics.

Consider just a few recent examples from my own community, the Lehigh Valley metropolitan area in eastern Pennsylvania. One Moravian congregation has made occasional visits to church partners in Tanzania and Nepal; another has sent groups to Haiti. A Methodist church sent a volunteer group to South Africa, while a different Methodist church has sent groups to Jamaica and Kenya. An individual member of a nondenominational Christian church arranged a trip on her own for other church members, working out the details with a Haitian pastor in nearby Philadelphia who has a church in Haiti.

Programs like these, publicized and organized locally, are nearly impossible to study in detail. The numbers are so vast that it is not possible to know their full scope. They have no NGO designation and very little Web presence. The sum total and impact of thousands of such volunteer efforts have yet to be measured, but they are certainly a very important part of the international volunteer phenomenon and deserve attention. They also raise concerns about impact, especially as many of the missions do not return to the same locations and may leave behind medications in communities and never follow up.

Robert Wuthnow writes about the constantly increasing global outreach on the part of American churches. He mentions many of the same factors influencing this growth that are outlined in the introduction for international volunteering activities more generally. Additionally, as congregations become more prosperous, more likely to include immigrants, and more exposed to the global economy and world travel, they increasingly devote resources to international mission activities. This is particularly true of the wealthy "megachurches," which engage heavily in evangelical activities.[8]

While almost all faith-based volunteering is located in Christian organizations, there are a few Jewish and Muslim groups. American Jewish World Service (AJWS) places volunteers with NGOs in developing countries on both short- and longer-term projects and provides financial support for many grassroots organizations. In accord with Jewish tradition, its volunteers do not promote their own religious views; their efforts center on the pursuit of global justice, and they integrate volunteer activities with a study of Jewish values to make volunteers more aware of their role as advocates for justice. Hillel: The Foundation for Jewish Campus Life partners with organizations such as the American Jewish Joint Distribution Committee and Repair the World to sponsor short-term trips with similar goals.[9] The Islamic Medical Association of North America (IMANA) also sends medical and nonmedical volunteers to a variety of countries to provide medical relief in times of disaster, and it offers training and other forms of development assistance in more than thirty countries worldwide.[10]

Not all faith-based organizations that sponsor short-term volunteer trips incorporate religious practice in their programs. There is, indeed, considerable variety in how religious faith informs the work of these organizations and of individual volunteers. I encountered three quite different approaches.

One is that religious faith or affiliation with a church community may motivate individuals to create or participate in overseas health programs, but these programs do not include any specific religious activity. Some call this "evangelism through action."[11] For example, Centura Health, a system representing both Catholic and Adventist hospitals, sends medical volunteers to many countries to support religious hospitals. Although this hospital system describes its mission as "extend[ing] the healing ministry of Christ,"[12] Greg Hodgson, Centura's global health director, explains that the organization's short-term missions are not intended to carry out any religious agenda. "As a faith-based organization here in Colorado," he says, "often when we have meetings, they'll start with a reflection. It's not necessarily worship or something like that, but it's just some thoughts to hopefully encourage people to think a little bit beyond just the immediate. We do those reflections also when we have these groups out [in other countries], just within our own group, but other than that, we don't get involved in any type of evangelistic or religious activities outside, so it's purely health care."

The second approach has organizations offering religious teaching and prayer when requested by local hosts or after their medical work is completed for the day; they are not purposely or directly integrated into the group's health-related activities. For example, the founder and codirector of a faith-based organization that sponsors health programs in two Caribbean nations told me, "We see our job as just to fulfill the Great Commission, which is to care for the poor and the lost. In the process of that, people ask about faith or to be prayed for, but we don't do evangelism. . . . The distinction we made was, if we're going out to a village to do a mobile clinic, I'm not going to make somebody sit there and listen to a sermon before they get seen."

She recounted an experience that led to the group's decision to keep any religious discussion separate from the medical work: "One day after I had been [in Haiti] three years, the Voudou priest came to my clinic. He had never come before. I had a dentist in and the priest had a bad tooth, and I said to him, 'This is the first time you ever came to the clinic. How come you never came to clinic?' He said, 'I came one time and they made me feel so bad out front with the sermon.' And I stopped it after that. He's a valuable person, too, right? I don't want to alienate him. If my job is to show the love of God to someone and I alienate them, how am I going to show them the love of God?"

Evangelical practices and preaching are integral or primary in the third approach. "As a Christian organization," one responding organization wrote, "sharing our purpose and message of salvation in Jesus is our major goal. However, we do desire to improve the health of the people in any area we serve. This is the right thing to do. We have helped pilot world-class health programs in some areas."

Even when proselytizing is not directly incorporated into the work, though, the religious basis for that work is often made quite obvious to patients. "None of us would be here without the conviction that Jesus calls us to love our neighbor and that our relationship with Jesus is primary in our life and ministry," reads an e-mail sent by a physician who served in a mission hospital in Nepal. "The motto of the hospital is 'We serve, Jesus heals,' and we have seen wonderful examples of that. There is no proselytizing, but patients are given the opportunity to be prayed for and/or attend chapel services. I believe strongly that a good part of the problems of the country (not only poverty but also the general sense of hopelessness) is connected to the fatalism of Hinduism and that giving people life thru a knowledge of their Savior is part of our calling."

Some programs incorporate prayer directly into their health services. An American physician working full-time at a hospital in Niger explained, "We treat everyone, not just Christians. The staff will offer to pray with patients; they always ask before they pray and Muslims generally like this and very few people say no. While Muslim prayers are not encouraged, people are allowed to pray as long as where they set up their 'prayer circles' does not block the flow of traffic."

Minister Mable Humphrey described the role of evangelism in her occasional mission trips:

> Our team includes pastors and licensed ministers, and we work the evangelism in the form of Bible study classes, health classes about our bodies, counseling and biblical leadership, and songs and games for the children. We attend churches in the evening after clinic; the pastors and ministers have a chance to teach or preach. Even the medical team members pray with the patients, and as we teach and explain medical procedures, we end the encounter with a word of hope. If times permits, we also go out into the communities and do hours of street ministry with singing and sermonettes. Whatever church and pastor we work with, we leave the new converts in their care to be discipled. So we work evangelism into our schedule every opportunity we get.

At the airport in Port-au-Prince, I spoke with departing volunteers from Georgia Baptists for Haiti, an organization run by the Georgia Baptist Convention that has "preach, teach, heal, build" as its slogan. Every week another group of volunteers goes to Haiti, where they staff clinics in several locations. This particular group had an ob-gyn, a nurse, and students who helped with triage and also prayed and preached with patients at the "preaching table" that sat between the doctor they had just seen and the pharmacy station that dispensed their medications. The campus minister accompanying the group told me that the patients are not working, so they have time to hear the Gospel. They are asked if they want to hear about God's work, and most agree. All agree to be prayed for, he recounted. An undergraduate nursing student was very enthusiastic about the experience. "I worked under a nurse practitioner," she told me. "It was great; God did good work."

At the medical missions conference described earlier, several speakers emphasized that medical care is a means for bringing Christianity and salvation to the people they treat and their family members, not a goal by itself. For example, a nurse who has worked on many short-term mission trips said, "A missionary in the context of God's mission is one who is sent to bring light into the dark world by sharing the gospel of Christ. . . . Jesus said, 'I will heal you and then I will tell you. . . . Meet people's needs first and then share the Gospel.' Feeding people and building wells, for example, are an avenue to the more important goal."

Other speakers concurred that medical care is primarily a means to the greater goal. One said, "The greatest injustice is not dying hungry or dying from illness. The greatest injustice is having those needs met and then going [to hell] for eternity."

A conference speaker explained that an important goal is to reach the THUMB people—Tribals, Hindus, Unreligious, Muslims, and Buddhists— and bring them the Gospel. A related concept among some missionary groups is "the 10/40 window"—the countries of Africa and Asia between ten and forty degrees latitude north of the equator, in which there are very few Christians. Many of these countries do not admit Christian missionaries, so organizations have taken to gaining "creative access," using medical care as an entrée.[13] Medical Missions Response, which sends volunteers to countries in the 10/40 window, has this goal: "As God has gifted us with health care skills, we will use this tool, under His guidance and direction, to take the Gospel to the unreached peoples of the world. Using their professional skills, representatives of MMR endeavor to cross all barriers and open doors for the Gospel so that all people groups may have access to salvation."[14]

These views on the primacy of the religious mission are reflected as well in a handbook for medical missionaries, in which the authors write,

> Your overriding motivation for the trip must be that you have realized that God has called you and your family to provide service to the Lord, the missionaries on the field, and the hurting people surrounding them. You are going to try to communicate in whatever way you can that Jesus Christ is Lord and He has saved you personally. . . . Remember that medicine per se is NOT the raison d'être for your being there nor for the hospital's existence. The basic goal of medical missions is evangelism. Present Jesus Christ to patients, their families, and their friends. . . . Many patients and family members come to know Christ as they see the loving care and integrate it with the messages they hear during the ward visits and services. A medical cure has an effect of less than 70 years; a spiritual cure for the uniformly fatal disease of sin is eternal in its effect.[15]

When I asked an open-ended question about organizational goals, 40 percent of the participants who identified their groups as faith-based acknowledged missionary work as one of the top four priorities; the other 60 percent did not mention it. In the survey distributed to Catholic Health

Association member hospitals and health systems, participants were asked what they considered the three most important goals of international medical missions and were offered thirteen possible responses. Some 22 percent of people who had organized trips in the previous five years selected "carrying out missionary work" as one of the top goals.[16]

These results suggest that for the majority of established faith-based organizations that sponsor overseas medical missions quite regularly, missionary goals are not a primary consideration. However, since there is very little information about the occasional missions sponsored by thousands of individual churches, it is impossible to know for sure how widespread evangelizing might be in those programs.

Religious faith motivates many people to sacrifice themselves to serve others, and religious institutions provide vast numbers of people in poor communities around the world with healthcare services, services that are often not available otherwise. Host communities that have long ago converted to Christianity often welcome the solidarity and support of coreligionists from other countries.[17]

Still, medical volunteering through religious organizations has a somewhat troubling history and a legacy that continues to raise questions. It has long been associated with colonial conquest and the imposition of Western institutions and values in other parts of the world.[18] Today's medical missions are also problematic, particularly when medical care is treated as a means to achieving the primary goal of evangelizing. Not only is tying services to prayer and preaching potentially coercive, but health programs sponsored by faith-based organizations may exclude vital services—such as contraception— because of religious objections.

Short-term health volunteering cannot be studied properly without a focus on the diverse activities and purposes of faith-based missions that dominate the field and continue to grow and devote billions of U.S. dollars to this purpose.[19]

NGOs—Growing Like Crazy

Half of all volunteer-sponsoring organizations are not faith-based. They are, in order of numbers in the international volunteering world, NGOs, educational institutions, and corporations. But the boundaries between these types are somewhat loose. Indeed, many university and health professions students who participate in international volunteer programs do so through NGOs, not through their own schools. And many NGOs rely on recruitment through student "chapters" and social networks for large numbers of their volunteers. Corporations that sponsor health missions overseas often do so in collaboration with NGOs and/or universities. Nevertheless, each of these sectors has a unique history and set of priorities when it organizes short-term volunteer trips.

During the past few decades of huge cutbacks in publicly funded safety nets in the poorer countries, we have seen an increase in the number of international development agencies and a tremendous proliferation of localized NGOs based in both wealthy and poor countries. They promote volunteering as a way to fill the gaps created by these cutbacks as well as by chronic lack of health services and infrastructure in much of the world.

While faith-based organizations are, technically, also nonprofit, nongovernmental organizations, the label "NGO" is typically reserved for non-faith-based nonprofits (and that is how I use it in this book). NGOs are fewer in number in the medical volunteering world than the religious groups, range from one-person operations to large and widely recognized groups, and send more volunteers on average than the faith-based organizations.

As of September 2015, the Union of International Associations Yearbook lists more than 68,000 international (i.e., operating in more than one country) NGOs and intergovernmental organizations (IGOs). It adds about 1,200 new organizations to the list annually.[20]

The increase in small and often specialized NGOs creates more opportunities for the volunteers on whom these groups rely to achieve their goals.[21] And they serve a purpose for governments, too. As one researcher has observed, "An NGO is an efficient tool with which to harvest donor money. Rich governments have lost their appetite for handing over checks to poor, corrupt, and dictatorial regimes. So they hand them to NGOs instead."[22] This idea is confirmed by other researchers: "Driven in some measure by donor preferences, the number of NGOs worldwide ballooned during the 1990s from 6000 to 26,000. . . . Overall aid funding to nonstate organizations from major donors such as the World Bank and European bilateral agencies grew 350% between 1990 and 1999."[23]

Often it is individuals who start these groups, part of a movement sometimes called "social entrepreneurship" designed to address social problems through private efforts.[24] It is indeed a worldwide phenomenon. In Ghana it seemed that half the people I met—including a taxi driver, a minister, and a college professor—had all started their own NGOs for different health and educational projects.

In addition to the small NGOs, several major private foundations have emerged since the 1990s that also served to shift the emphasis in global health away from public to private efforts. The best known are the Bill and Melinda Gates Foundation, started in 1994, and the William J. Clinton Foundation, established in 2001.

NGOs constitute the most dynamic sector in the international volunteering world, a space in which passionate and talented individuals can identify a problem and mobilize people and money to address it. Some well-known organizations that sponsor international volunteers, such as Unite for Sight, and hundreds—probably thousands—of smaller ones were founded by individual college students, physicians, or business people, with an idea for something that needed to be done and the drive and ability to make it happen.[25]

Dr. Gary Morsch is one such individual. He founded Heart to Heart International (HHI) in Olathe, Kansas, in 1992 in response to the critical needs for medication and supplies in Russia after the collapse of the Soviet Union. Working through his local Rotary Club and with donations from pharmaceutical and other companies, he flew to Russia on a U.S. Air Force-supplied cargo plane to distribute the supplies. Thus HHI began its activities with onetime visits (or the shipping of relief supplies) to places identified as needing emergency assistance. These include tornado-damaged towns in the United States and locations such as those in the Philippines destroyed by a 2013 typhoon.[26]

HHI's focus on disaster relief continues to this day. Almost immediately after the devastating earthquake struck Haiti in 2010, Dr. Morsch flew into the capital to provide emergency services. This was a major turning point for HHI; the organization decided to remain in Haiti, unlike many other groups that stayed only temporarily and have sometimes been accused of causing great harm.[27]

Like Dr. Morsch, Dr. Chuck Dietzen—founder of Timmy Global Health, an NGO based in Indianapolis, Indiana, that sends medical "brigades" to Ecuador, Dominican Republic, and Guatemala—was inspired by his own experience in service to create a new organization. Both had worked with Mother Teresa in Calcutta.

Despite such inspiring examples, NGOs based in the United States and in Europe have been subjected to growing criticism for the work they do in poorer countries. A group of authors at Health Alliance International, a Seattle-based NGO affiliated with the University of Washington, wrote a "Code of Conduct" for NGOs titled "Strengthening Health Systems in Poor Countries."[28] In it, they contend that the involvement of international organizations and volunteers in the health services of poor countries leads to increased fragmentation of services, management burden on local health managers (as they must respond to many different organizations with separate programs), brain drain from public-sector services to NGOs (which often pay higher salaries and offer desirable training opportunities), and myriad projects that collapse when NGO grant funding ends.

"Driven by donor demands," the authors contend, "NGOs often focus narrowly on vertical programs that serve limited populations in confined geographical settings for single health problems. As a result, NGOs frequently create showcase projects with questionable sustainability and perfunctory linkages to local health services."[29]

Jim Butcher and Peter Smith, two English researchers, voice a similar concern in their study of volunteer tourism. "The personal element [offered by NGOs] appears positive—it bypasses big government and eschews big business. Yet it also bypasses the democratic imperative of representative government and reduces development to individual acts of charity."[30]

Linda Polman's critique of the role of NGOs is particularly sharp. In her book *The Crisis Caravan: What's Wrong with Humanitarian Aid?* the freelance Dutch journalist focuses on disaster and war zones, where NGOs and international organizations congregate and compete—not always with the best results. She recounts stories of NGOs appearing in refugee camps with U.S. medical students, who then proceed to carry out procedures they aren't licensed to perform back home, and of surgeons who visit briefly and provide no aftercare in case of complications.[31]

Polman's work addresses several of the problems identified in this book, and she adds some provocative insights into the proliferation of small NGOs—in particular, ones she describes as having been started by entrepreneurial individuals in response to their *own* sense of what needs to be done, and that she calls "MONGOs," for "My Own NGOs." It is the past failures of international aid organizations that are responsible, in part, for the growth of these MONGOs by individuals who hope to do better.

"MONGOs make up what has become a vast countermovement, run by people who are convinced they can get things sorted out in a crisis zone more effectively, quickly, and cheaply than the 'real' aid workers with—to MONGO eyes at least—self-serving motives and cumbrous bureaucracy."[32]

Joanne Carman and Rebecca Nesbit studied NGOS in North Carolina and noted some related concerns.[33] They asked why the organizations were started, and most founders told them they thought they were responding to an unmet need in the community. Yet very few had formally assessed these needs; rather, they tended to be passionate individuals who "just knew" based on their personal or work experience, or who had "asked around." More than half had no experience working or volunteering for a nonprofit organization; some, the researchers indicate, apparently started their organization at least in part to provide themselves with employment doing something they love. These organizations tended to be small and to work independently instead of collaborating with the larger nonprofit sector.

The dominance of NGOs in the policy and services of many low-income countries has raised serious concerns. As journalists Klarreich and Polman write, "Critics have taken to calling these LDCs [less developed countries] 'NGO Republics'—countries where nongovernmental organizations and wealthy donor entities have created parallel states endlessly richer and, at the end of the day, more powerful than the national governments themselves. Ultimately, it's the NGOs that decide how these governments will spend the funds and run their countries, to the tune of tens of billions of dollars a year."[34]

NGOs represent a complex stew of remarkable energy and dedication to improving the lives of poor people combined with a mixed record of accomplishment. The creation of thousands of individual projects focused on specific places or diseases or body parts (eyes, shoulders, mouths, etc.) can make a difference in those circumstances but exacerbate the fragmentation of services and the problem of lack of accountability. Thus the benefits and the risks are both large.

Schools and Students

Today, nearly every college and university, at least in the United States, has invested in building its profile in global studies and international activities. Study-abroad programs, international service learning, overseas internships, and exchange programs are expanding everywhere. Some of these are a response to student demand rooted in their interest in community service, which has become widely popular in schools; some high schools even require a certain number of community service hours for graduation. The programs are also a direct reflection of the increasingly common view among individual students, undergraduate and graduate: there is value in obtaining international experiences for "the development of a range of values, knowledges, skills and attitudes that are aligned with and in part equip young people to compete more effectively in increasingly transnationalised skilled worker labour markets."[35]

For many students and their mentors, international volunteering is perceived as an important part of career preparation in the globalized world, although employers may not always recognize this.[36] But beyond what is learned, just going on a volunteer trip has increasingly become a way to stand out with admissions officers and in the competition for jobs. Personal status is surely part of the picture. As one organizer told me, "Students are especially trying to figure out ways to separate themselves from the pack. Everybody goes to London and gets drunk . . . but not everybody works on water systems in Tanzania."

Among college students, all kinds of volunteering have become more commonplace. An analysis of four nationally representative cohorts of college students from the National Postsecondary Student Aid Study showed an increase in the percentage of students who reported that service was required by their study program, but these students represented small percentages of all those who performed services (which increased from 39% in 1996 to 47% in 2008).[37]

Onetime service, often in response to a specific crisis, is generally voluntary rather than required as part of a study program. It, too, has grown among American youth, from 9 percent in 2000 to 25 percent in 2008. Some observers believe this may be related in part to Americans' desire to do something for others immediately following dramatic events, such as the 9/11 attacks, Hurricane Katrina, and the Haitian earthquake.[38]

One study proposes another explanation for increased international service: first-generation American students wanting to give back to the less privileged, often in their families' countries of origin.[39] So far there is not enough information about this particular phenomenon, although it seems likely and can be seen in examples cited in this book of Syrian American physicians working in refugee camps and Haitian Americans participating in missions to their home country.

Another very important driver of growing student involvement in volunteering is the globalization of universities and health professions. Many new global studies programs require students to participate in international experiences.[40] "International service," write Amanda Moore McBride and Eric Mlyn, "is but just one small part of this broader trend where U.S. universities are opening satellite campuses in Asia and the Middle East, creating partnerships and collaborations with institutions across the globe, and sending more of our students around the world."[41] These include growing numbers of students who study abroad.

At the undergraduate level, several NGOs promote opportunities for students to spend a week or more in medical overseas missions. Global Medical Training, Timmy Global Health, Unite for Sight, and many others develop campus-based chapters as a basis for organizing students to learn about global health, raise money for programs, and recruit students for volunteer trips.

There is enormous demand from students for short-term overseas programs, says the director of Global Education and Study Abroad at a large state university.

> We are seeing [prospective] medical students, for example, the first question they ask is, "How am I going to go abroad in my program?" "How am I going to pay for medical school?" is only the second question. We're seeing this with applicants and we're seeing it with the students once they arrive. At least 70 to 75 percent are asking that question and they're quite serious about it. It's a question to which we're very challenged to respond. Virtually everyone wants to go to a developing country, particularly Africa, to a certain extent Latin America. . . . There's the whole medical Spanish, medical culture and Hispanic cultures acquisition piece, and that's something that a lot of students are interested in . . . being prepared to serve . . . what they perceive as an important patient constituency [at home].

If the main goal is to learn how to relate to Latino immigrants in one's home community, it does seem that working in that community and taking an intensive Spanish course could better achieve this. Spending $2,000 to hang out for a week with other Americans and work in clinics in a Latin American country where the patients may not even speak Spanish but rather an indigenous language such as Kichwa is hardly the best way to achieve that goal. But there are obviously other attractions.

Dr. Neal Nathanson, former associate dean for Global Health Programs at the University of Pennsylvania School of Medicine, concurs that the increase in creation of university-based global health programs results from student demand. Recounting how his own position was created, he explains that student insistence drove a great deal of the growth in programs. "The impetus for a new program in global health came from medical students starting a group. The dean wanted the medical students out of his office; they were [there] demanding programs."

This phenomenon is hardly limited to U.S. universities. One 2009 review of international health electives at medical schools in the United Kingdom found that each year U.K. medical students alone spend the equivalent of 350 years' time in developing countries![42]

Health professional schools of all kinds—medicine, nursing, public health, and dentistry—have greatly increased their offerings in response to student demand. The International Federation of Medical Students, which represents 1.2 million medical students from ninety-one countries, is one of many organizations voicing this demand; the group "openly calls for medical schools to ensure a comprehensive global health framework within their curriculum. Universities, and their medical education and training programs, are hurrying to keep pace with the demand."[43] Institutions believe they will be more attractive to potential students and donors alike by developing such programs.[44]

This is one striking example of how organizational priorities and needs (or an individual dean's desire both to please students and to keep them out of his office) are driving the development of short-term medical volunteering programs. Students who can afford to spend the money for such trips pressure institutions to create opportunities, subsidize them, and sometimes offer credit as well. They expect to gain even more career advantages in the process, giving them an extra leg up by comparison with students who have fewer personal resources. But there is little research to answer whether the host community benefits in this scenario.

The Prevalence of Electives Abroad among Medical Students

According to an online 2008 survey of 96 U.S. medical schools, 11 percent had a global health track for students, 45 percent offered opportunities to perform preclinical research abroad, 61 percent offered international opportunities over school holidays, and 87 percent had international clinical electives. These numbers have surely increased since.

A 2009 survey of American surgical residents found that 92 percent wanted an international experience; 82 percent gave it higher priority than other kinds of electives. And a 2010 study noted that medical student participation in global health electives had jumped from 6 percent in 1994 to 31 percent in 2011 and that 52 percent of residencies offered a global health elective. (McKinley et al. 2008; Nelson 2012, 184; Powell 2009.)

Some short-term student service trips are coordinated through a central office at the school, but many students travel overseas on their own or in groups organized by individual faculty or students. Many individual students have started their own NGOs for a vast array of purposes and recruited others to participate, but the schools do not typically sponsor these. Faculty may involve students in their research or have contacts willing to help arrange for students to have a good experience in their countries.

Programs for graduate students in health professions are particularly active in providing hands-on experience. The institutions often get support from a variety of groups such as the Association of American Medical Colleges, Global Health Education Consortium, American Medical Student Association, Foundation for Advancement of International Medical Education and Research, and Consortium of Universities for Global Health, all of which have played an important role in fostering programs in health professional schools.[45]

The University of Pennsylvania offers a useful model for preparing and mentoring graduate students for international experiences. Many U.S. educational institutions have developed global health programs in recent years, but UPenn's program is unusual in that it fosters collaboration among multiple professional schools, including public health, nursing, medicine, and dentistry. These schools share a core course in global health and sometimes participate in common overseas programs, but each one also offers different types of experiences.

Dr. Marjorie Muecke, Global Health Director in the School of Nursing at the time of our interview, describes the approach in her school. "There are two types of short-term study-abroad programs that nursing students at the University of Pennsylvania can take—observation only and hands on, or engaging in clinical practice. Both are part of elective courses that involve an academic portion before going abroad or while there. In addition, several Penn Nursing faculty take master's program students (all of whom are RNs) to Haiti to provide patient care—these experiences are not for academic credit. While they are there, they also coach local healthcare providers."

In response to student demands for opportunities, many colleges and health profession schools contract with intermediary organizations to make all the arrangements for students to have overseas experiences. Amizade, an NGO based in Pittsburgh, Pennsylvania, for example, offers a variety of services ranging from connecting students and schools with community organizations in other countries to managing semester-abroad programs—including curricula, logistics, and community placements—to placing nursing students and medical residents in clinics where the group has partnership arrangements.

Brandon Blache-Cohen, Amizade's executive director, explains how the group works with schools:

> Our mission is to empower individuals and communities to worldwide service, so we're looking at community interest and needs and student interest and needs and we have the luxury to be able to not just focus on students, which I think a lot of colleges and universities are fixated on.
>
> [Health professional schools are] a huge growth area for us. We're now working with West Virginia University's medical school. We have run nursing programs from a couple of different universities. We've worked

with pharmacy schools as well. But the big thing that we're interested in is medical rotations that we're doing now in Brazil. We have a really interesting partnership with a clinic that we've been working with for 18 years now, but it's progressed to the point now where we're comfortable bringing doctors and dentists who have been practicing for years to work with the community there.

The criticism of premedical and medical student involvement in short-term trips is increasing, with many publications examining the common practices under which students are allowed to interact with patients in ways that would never be allowed in their home countries.[46] These criticisms are producing some changes, including the development of national guidelines and efforts to provide more rigorous preparation. For example, the University of Minnesota has developed "Global Ambassadors for Patient Safety," a required online program that emphasizes what untrained students going abroad should and should not be doing in patient care situations. The University's motto, according to Tricia Todd of the Health Careers Center, is "If you can't do it here, you shouldn't do it there."

Another indicator of change: I spoke at a global health conference in 2014 about short-term volunteering and mentioned the resume-building motivations some students emphasize. A medical school admissions committee member in the audience commented that a short volunteer trip is now considered a red flag. His committee looks at how applicants talk about such programs, not only in their applications but also even in Facebook posts, with a skeptical eye toward those who lack a serious approach and understanding of their experience.

Corporate Volunteering

Just as colleges and universities have expanded their international service activities and NGOs have increased in numbers, private corporations now undertake more service activities that sometimes include promoting overseas volunteering. The rise in what is referred to as "corporate social responsibility" has led to a growing involvement of corporate groups in volunteer activities around the world, including in health-related missions.

Sarah Hayes, director of the Global Corporate Volunteer Council and formerly of the KPMG accounting firm, recounts some of the historical and organizational factors that have led companies to invest in volunteer efforts, especially since the late 1980s. "There was sort of a groundswell, partly coming from the "Thousand Points of Light" speech by then President George H. W. Bush . . . and even some societal things, I think, that were happening, the way the jobs world was changing and people were not necessarily staying from cradle to grave with one company, so looking at ways of enticing valuable employees to stay was part of the thinking. A whole bunch of factors kind of came together, and companies really wanted to look a little bit more at how they could be more involved in the community, be more responsive to community needs and relate to their employees' interests as well."

KPMG's direct involvement was particularly apparent in San Francisco. "We were dealing with the AIDS issue in a big, big way," Hayes continues, "and KPMG had a number of people who were HIV positive, and people were grappling with how to deal with that, and I think that pushed us along, too, perhaps."

In addition to the personal links, Hayes says there were business reasons.

> And also the reputational value, of course, as well, because some companies were not experiencing very good ones. So I think all of that coming together. People are very community minded, and coming out of universities they've been doing community work, they care about it, they have some kind of passion for bettering the world, and they know, it's not a secret anymore, they know that companies do this stuff. If they don't see that you have it, it may not be a deal breaker, if it's the perfect job, but it could be if all else is equal. Corporate social responsibility is a huge topic, which covers so many things, not just volunteering, but it is something that is increasingly important to all companies these days.

Corporations may organize their own service trips, but much more commonly they support employees' service more indirectly. Many companies have award programs for volunteers, give time off for service, and support fundraising for international service projects. Pharmaceutical companies are particularly active. For instance, Pfizer sponsors a Global Health Fellows Program that places its employees with development organizations for short-term assignments to "transfer their professional medical and business expertise in ways that promote access, quality and efficiency of health services for people in greatest need."[47] In 2011, Eli Lilly & Company announced the launch of "Lilly Ambassadors," a volunteer program for its employees with immediate plans to send groups of eight or nine ambassadors to different countries in Asia, Africa, and Central and South America for two-week service trips designed to "observe and assist" local health professionals and teachers.[48]

Microsoft offers another example of corporate support for international volunteering. One goal of the volunteer trip to Ecuador sponsored by Timmy Global Health in which I participated was to launch a program for electronic medical records to be used in the Amazon Basin. Several Microsoft employees who had worked on the program went to Ecuador to introduce and test it. One of them sponsored a poker tournament to raise funds for the trip, and Microsoft matched what was raised. Microsoft also pays organizations on a list of approved philanthropies for the time employees spend volunteering, at a rate of $17 an hour. Thus, between matching the tournament take and paying Timmy for a half dozen or so employees' time in Ecuador, there was a substantial corporate donation.

Many other companies donate medications and supplies to relief organizations such as Direct Relief International and Heart to Heart International, which use them in particular for crisis situations such as natural disasters. This could be considered an example of what has been called "cause-related marketing," the "association of a for-profit company with a non-profit organization with the intention of increasing the interest of both parties." CRM is intended to strengthen a company's image and expand its market while demonstrating its social responsibility and benefiting the nonprofit partner. Often, a company will market a particular product or brand in conjunction with a social cause.[49]

Occasionally a company directly sponsors an international volunteer trip, and Becton Dickinson (BD), a Fortune 500 multinational corporation that manufactures medical supplies, laboratory equipment, and diagnostic products, has pioneered in this regard. Its programs are described in chapter 2, which considers the different models sponsoring organizations adopt for their activities in the global health arena. Type of sponsorship is important in understanding the history and goals and problems surrounding specific volunteer efforts. But all types of sponsors can organize the wide range of programs that take volunteers to work in global health projects.

2

The Activities and Goals of Sponsoring Organizations

Types of Volunteer Trips

Regardless of the type of sponsorship, international volunteer trips differ considerably in length, frequency of visits, and activities. Short-term medical trips fall roughly into four types:

- One-shot or occasional visits for primary care, health education, or training
- One-shot or occasional visits for surgical intervention
- Periodic but regular visits to the same locations for screening and primary care
- Year-round operations with frequent short-term volunteers providing support for local professionals

The same organization may have multiple models, depending on the program or the country. Some combine health work with other projects such as church building, orphanage visits, or construction. When asked about the primary activities of volunteers, organizers most frequently cited direct provision of medical care (84%), health education (72%), and training of local health care workers (67%). Fewer than half mentioned environmental or sanitation improvements, needs assessment, constructing or rehabilitating buildings, public health research, and medical research.

One-shot or occasional visits for primary care, health education, or training may be the most common type of volunteer program, one that often involves untrained volunteers. Forty-four percent of organizations indicated that at least some of their volunteers participate in one-shot programs.

Mable Humphrey is a retired nurse and part-time pastor at a Baptist church in Bethlehem, Pennsylvania. She has a great deal of voluntary overseas medical mission experience, beginning with trips to Liberia that resulted in the creation of a clinic. In recent years, she has organized and led volunteer trips to Haiti. She does this as an individual, with some support from her own congregation, but essentially recruits, trains, and establishes partnerships on her own. Through a contact with a Haitian pastor and in collaboration with a representative of Haiti's Ministry of Health, Humphrey has organized a group from her church for several one-week annual visits to Haiti. The group includes a few trained medical personnel, pastors, and laypeople. One advantage is that among the volunteers are Haitian Americans who are very helpful in orienting the others to the culture and language.

The group has had a full agenda for their week: they organize a clinic in one community, for which they bring medications and medical supplies; they spend time in a school and an orphanage, and they hold prayer and Bible sessions with a church. Although they leave medications behind with the partner minister, the visit is not part of a continuous form of medical care. Volunteers express concerns about not being able to meet the expectations of the patients who flock to the clinic on the few days they are there.

Becton Dickinson has been involved in international volunteering for a decade—and offers a different example. Its motto is "Helping all people live healthy lives," and BD regularly donates medical supplies to humanitarian relief organizations. One volunteer program involves employees in providing laboratory training and support for American efforts against HIV/AIDS, primarily in African countries through the U.S. President's Emergency Plan for AIDS Relief program (PEPFAR).[1]

The annual Volunteer Service Trip, begun in 2005, includes about a dozen company employees selected from BD offices in different countries who are sent to one location to work on a variety of projects, including establishing laboratories and training laboratory workers, providing additional hands for primary care, community health training, and constructing facilities. Unlike most volunteers who make these kinds of trips, the BD participants are paid their normal salaries, and all their expenses are covered for the three-week trip.

A different group of BD volunteers worked each year for three years in Zambia, a period followed by three trips to Ghana and then Haiti. In each country, BD partnered with an American NGO with local programs or contacts. Through these collaborations, the volunteers participated in or supplemented ongoing programs or created one-time projects. The three BD service trips to Ghana involved working at clinics in different parts of the country, building housing for patient families at one clinic, setting up a laboratory, and training midwives. For the trips to Haiti, one team composed of nurses worked in regularly scheduled clinics to assist the Haitian physicians and staff; others did construction on volunteer facilities, and two groups developed and carried out one-week training programs for community health workers and laboratory workers.

Haiti, 2012. The main transport vehicle that takes volunteers and supplies to the clinics is affectionately referred to as "the cage," since it does look like one. The flatbed of a truck is enclosed in fencing, and along each side is a narrow bench where we sit; underneath and between the benches are boxes and bins of supplies. We volunteers are the odd creatures inside the cage as it bumps up and down the streets of Haiti's capital. There are a couple of narrow, slanting steps leading into the back of the truck but nothing to hold on to for helping to climb in except a piece of knotted rope hanging from the roof. So one at a time we grab the rope, pull ourselves up the steps, and land inside the cage. It takes what seems like two hours to go the fairly short distance from the volunteer center to the clinic, but it does give us our first real chance to look at some of Port-au-Prince.

The biggest challenge comes with needing a bathroom. The one in the pharmacy area is semiflooded, so we get to use the one in the school area downstairs, but wish we had not since there is no flush, and especially in the heat it is quite unpleasant. I learn an important lesson: an interesting challenge each day is to stay hydrated enough to prevent headaches and other problems but not so much as to need a bathroom.

Otherwise the clinic is pretty comfortable, probably because there is some breeze and plenty of seating. The laboratory, which had been built and equipped by previous volunteers from Becton Dickinson, is enclosed and air-conditioned and well stocked. There is no electricity in the neighborhood, we are told, so everything runs by generator. Some volunteers help the Haitian nurses as they see patients in the triage area and then send them to consult with the Haitian doctor in a closed office; patients then go to other rooms as needed for tests and/ or medications. There are not as many patients as expected, and the volunteers don't feel especially useful today.

After a few hours, we climb back onto the cage and return to the volunteer center in an upper-class neighborhood. There are three cooks, the food is good, and the electricity and Wi-Fi are pretty regular. And there is a delightful swimming pool. Not all volunteer trips experience such luxury, but after a hot day no one is complaining.

The next morning we depart at 6:30, taking the cage and a pickup truck. We head up the narrow mountain road to Fondwa, a village spread out over the hillside, and while it is remote and looks sparsely populated, it has an active "peasant association," a convent that before the earthquake ran a school and clinic, and even a university. Heart to Heart International is in this location because it was contacted by the Sisters of Charity in Kansas after the quake asking if the group could contact the convent in Fondwa and find out whether the nuns were OK. HHI was able to get there and report back to Kansas that the nuns were safe but that everything had been destroyed by the quake. With help from the Jewish Joint Distribution Committee and in partnership with the peasant association, HHI began to rebuild.

HHI brings volunteers to Fondwa once a week to see patients in what they call their "clinic in a can." This is a shipping container converted into a clinic, with separate rooms for patient exams, a laboratory, and a pharmacy. HHI workers brought this clinic on a flatbed truck up the mountain over roads that were in terrible condition and also had to bring a crane to lift the clinic off the flatbed and onto the ground. Eventually they stopped when they could go no farther, and that is where they set up the clinic, not far from the convent. The clinic is staffed by sisters who are nurses, but one day a week an HHI staff doctor goes there as well.

There are about sixty people waiting on benches under the shade of a tarp. Two sisters are there with patient folders, and each waiting patient has a form for today's visit that will go into the folder when he or she gets to the doctor. The forms have their names and ages.

The Haitian doctor who works for HHI quickly sets up in one of the rooms, and a volunteer nurse sets up in the pharmacy in another room. Two volunteers set up a table for triage, with two translators. They ask each person to state his or her chief complaints, then record temperature, blood pressure, pulse, and weight. I help with weight and temperature but have to convert each time to metric measurements, which is slow and confusing. Patients speak of weakness, dizziness, pains of various kinds. Some of the children look quite ill. Several people arrive on the backs of motorcycles while we are there, including an older woman with a crutch and another woman who is in great pain and distress and is seen ahead of the waiting people, who do not protest. After going through triage, they wait to see the doctor, which is of course a longer wait, and after the doctor, they take prescriptions to the pharmacy. It takes many hours to go through all the steps for what are ultimately sixty-five people, children and adults.

Then back to the volunteer center in the capital. Being here with a large group feels a little like being back in summer camp, in a really nice way. People are sharing rooms, mostly with bunk beds, eating together, and getting to know each other. It is a very impressive group. They have a high level of professionalism as well as great agility in adapting to unknown situations very quickly and a generosity of heart seen in how they all jump to help each other, whether it be in the clinic or over dinner.

With experience, BD's Volunteer Service Trips have come to offer more of the very continuity so crucial to program success. For example, Haitians who received laboratory and community health training were given a subsequent round of training to build on what they had learned in previous years. There has also been a greater effort to match services to country needs. In training laboratory workers, BD and Heart to Heart International have worked closely with the Haiti Ministry of Health and the National Laboratory in advance of the volunteer visits to determine the best way to plan training sessions. The training curriculum was developed through a four-way collaboration among the National Laboratory, BD, HHI, and Partners in Health (PIH) and was piloted in two weeklong sessions for PIH laboratory technicians taught by three BD volunteers. On the basis of this experience, BD and HHI further adapted the curriculum for the three training sessions carried out several months later in three locations around the country.

One-shot or occasional visits for surgical intervention are the least likely to involve untrained students or laypeople. One example is Prevention International—No Cervical Cancer (PINCC), established in 2005 by Dr. Kay Taylor, a gynecologist, following a medical mission to Honduras during which she saw more cases of women dying of cervical cancer than she had seen in her entire career. PINCC deals only with cervical cancer, and its visits are infrequent. It works in Africa, Latin America, and India, using its resources to screen for and treat cervical cancer and train others to do the same. In particular, local physicians are trained to carry out LEEP (loop electrosurgical excision procedure) to remove abnormal tissue. PINCC also provides health education and equips facilities; thus it has a multifaceted but sporadic approach to a single disease. Unlike many volunteer organizations, it focuses on trained medical personnel, rather than students, as volunteers.

John Adams, administrative director of PINCC-India and a retired business professor, tells a fairly typical story of how a series of coincidences and personal contacts and history led to a program in that country.

> My wife and I have been going for many years to an ashram in southern India for spiritual study, and that ashram has five hospitals. My wife worked in the gynecology clinic and would see two to four cases of cervical cancer a week. She only actually saw one cervical cancer case in her entire thirty-year practice in San Francisco, because with Pap smears and all that, we've learned how to prevent it.
>
> She started looking around and found that [Dr. Kay Taylor,] a woman she had been a resident with thirty years ago . . . had already set up [PINCC]. [Taylor] was developing protocols for screening and treating and training local physicians to do it, because it's basically a capacity-building program. We went with [PINCC] on a mission to Kenya and Tanzania and learned the process. I did everything from registering patients to washing speculums in a washtub out in the sun outside the school. My wife was inside doing pelvic exams on a school desk.

The creation of PINCC programs in a few locations in India is an excellent example of how individual encounters can result in programs their founders never anticipated. As Adams continues,

We heard about the ashram's mobile hospital, which goes out and visits a different village the first twelve days of each month. Each village is a magnet village for up to twenty other villages, so there were 250,000 people with access to free world-class health care living in remote, poor villages in southern India. It's a comprehensive daylong clinic, basically that has orthopedics and pediatrics and obstetrics and light surgery. They even can make a full set of dentures in one day. The director of that mobile hospital got instantly what we were doing and got very excited about it.

[Now] Mysore medical college has invited us to create a curriculum. They say we are a big enough medical school that if we can make this work in our curriculum, we can get the national medical board to mandate HPV and cervical cancer education in all of the schools.

PINCC's visits are sporadic and occasionally do not come off as planned for a variety of bureaucratic and logistical reasons. But the goal of equipping facilities and training staff members is designed to keep the program going without outside volunteers. The focus on one disease only is similar to that of many programs around the world that select malaria or river blindness or specific anatomic malformations (cleft palate in many countries, undeveloped ears in Ecuador, child colorectal anomalies in Ghana and China). Such programs have been criticized for fragmenting care and staffs while creating excessive demands on local health officials; PINCC-India attempts to avoid this problem by working through the existing mobile clinic outreach.

Colorectal Team Overseas (CTO) is based at Cincinnati Children's Hospital and operates under the hospital's nonprofit status. Since 2008, a team of about thirty colorectal surgeons, anesthesiologists, nurses, and other volunteers has traveled about once each year to do surgery for children born with anorectal malformations and to train others in their treatment. Led by Dr. Marc Levitt, a pediatric colorectal surgeon at the hospital, the team has worked in Honduras, Ethiopia, Ghana, and South Africa. On each trip, several dozen children have had operations, and the team has trained local surgeons in how to do the specialized surgery required.

"I went to Honduras with a surgical organization," Dr. Levitt told me, explaining how the group got started, "and I didn't like the way they operated, without a proper ICU and medications. So I started my own project. Smile Train [an NGO that sends surgical missions around the world to perform cleft palate and cleft lip repairs and train local professionals to perform the surgeries] sponsored one of my trips because of their interest in sustainability by training. They sent e-mails to their partners around the world who are plastic surgeons asking if they needed colorectal help and got over one hundred responses. That made me realize I had to go out to the world because they aren't going to be able to come to Cincinnati."

Surgeons from other parts of the world also visit Cincinnati on occasion to train with Dr. Levitt's group there, and they are often the ones who host CTO's visits to their home countries. Dr. Levitt's aim is to continue to find new sites rather than to return to countries that CTO has already visited. The continuity of support is provided from a distance, primarily by e-mail.

Timmy Global Health, introduced briefly in chapter 1, offers an interesting model for *periodic but regular visits to the same locations for screening and primary care*. Based in Indianapolis, Indiana, the NGO was founded in 1997 by Dr. Charles Dietzen ("Dr. Chuck"), a pediatric physical medicine and rehabilitation specialist. The group sends approximately four hundred volunteers per year—about one-third of them medical professionals and the others students and lay volunteers—on medical "brigades" to Ecuador, Guatemala, and the Dominican Republic. The organization is named for Dr. Chuck's older brother Timmy, who passed away in his infancy.

Timmy's medical and nonmedical volunteers work together in week-long brigades that circulate among the same communities every two to two and a half months. The timing depends to some extent on when students from Timmy chapters on American college campuses have breaks from class.

During a typical weeklong brigade in the Amazon Basin region, clinics are set up in different villages each day, generally at a community center. In the weeks beforehand, Timmy Global Health community workers and representatives from the local government circulate in the region to alert people that the clinic will be open and to sell the nominally priced tickets that must be presented upon arrival. At the clinic itself, patients can obtain medications and vitamins for no additional charge; volunteers also offer fluoride treatments for children and parasite prophylaxis.

Timmy's in-country practices are based on the premise that the same communities should be visited every two months or so to provide continuity of care to patients, including regular medication renewal. Explains Matt MacGregor, former executive director,

We have an ability to do chronic-care management, because we're returning to the same communities, so we see a lot of the same patients. Obviously,
we're not going to be there for two and a half months, so it's not perfect, but
there is clearly an attempt to deal with that major constraint of short-term
trips, which is that you're there and then you're gone. There's a continuity
aspect in that we have more accountability because we're in the communities more consistently. . . . If someone gets seriously ill from something we
gave them in one of our clinics, we'd know about it, because we're going to
go back to the same community in two and a half months.

Of course, having to wait months to return to the same village clinic
on the one day that the next Timmy brigade is due to arrive is not a
good solution for a person with complications. The fact that there is
a full-time Timmy staff member living in the region and continuous
relationships with a local hospital and Timmy community health workers offers the possibility for better follow-up than is available in the
one-shot programs. There are also public clinics in the region. But the
gaps are real.

Beyond providing primary care, Timmy is committed to referring patients needing more specialized care to partner hospitals. In Ecuador, for
example, Timmy staff members—both Ecuadorean and those from the
United States who live in the country—devote considerable time at the
end of each brigade to making sure patients from the clinics needing referrals get to the hospital even if it is far from their homes. As MacGregor
says, "In many cases, we provide transport or finance transport or pay for
translators for our indigenous patients or send a social worker to the hospital with them if they're afraid to go. We potentially bring in their family,
potentially show up at the hospital with them and help them through the
process if they can't read, those types of things. All in all, it's part of our
attempt to try and ensure that we do not just treat patients, but we support
them with other programming that helps them navigate often complicated
local health systems."

This distinguishes Timmy from other health NGOs; it is unusual to
place so much emphasis on a program of ongoing referral of patients who
need more specialized care and to provide support for their travel and
accommodations to make it successful. As we will see in a later chapter,
tracking the success of this referral system is a key element of Timmy
Global Health's assessment of its programs.

Timmy focuses almost entirely on primary care and referrals and occasionally organizes health education programs for community health workers, but in 2012 it sponsored a surgical brigade for hernia repairs in its partner hospital in the Amazon Basin. A surgeon who specializes in hernias happened to have visited the area on vacation and liked it, so he contacted Timmy and organized a brigade of other hernia specialists to return. Staff members from Timmy and its partner hospital collected referrals during their regular patient outreach, and in six days the visiting surgeons and Ecuadorian physicians and staff carried out sixty-eight operations.

Providing financial support for partners is another important part of Timmy's activities. "We help in financing partner organizations, hospitals, medical clinics, healthcare organizations that are working in the developing world," says MacGregor. "We do some financing of public health projects. Right now we finance a malnutrition project, a midwife training project, a community health worker training program. We donate money for their salaries and medicines and other needs. Not a ton of money, I'd love to improve it, but it's there."

Campus-based education is an additional aspect of the group's mission: Timmy's nonmedical volunteers come largely from the several dozen college campuses with "Timmy chapters" that work to involve students over several years in advocacy and educational activities to address health disparities in their local communities. Chapters also engage in fund-raising for Timmy's work in other countries and select the students who will get to participate in an overseas brigade.

Some organizations have *year-round operations with frequent short-term volunteers providing support for local professionals*. CURE International in Lemoyne, Pennsylvania, is a religious organization that provides surgical interventions for children. Founded in 1996 by Dr. Scott Harrison, an orthopedic surgeon and business executive, and his wife Sally, CURE has established a presence in more than twenty-seven countries, including hospitals in ten countries. At the group's website, its hospital in Niamey, Niger, is described this way: "CURE's hospital in Niger is the only one of its kind in the entire country, offering specialty surgical care for handicapped children with a variety of conditions. Located in the capital city of Niamey, the hospital attracts patients from every region of the country. With 2 operating theaters and 24 beds, our annual surgical capacity is approximately 1,000 and we typically see over 250 patients per month at our outpatient clinics. The Hospital has a total staff of 63 including 5 Expatriates."[2] The role of short-term volunteers in a hospital such as CURE in Niamey is to supplement the permanent staff members who care for children with occasional visiting groups of volunteer surgeons and other medical professionals.

Leron Lehman, an American who formerly was executive director of the hospital, explains. "We don't rely on volunteers for any day-to-day activities; we only use them to help us treat more patients, to provide training to our staff, or to fill in for a doctor who is away on leave. Nearly all of our volunteers are medical professionals that come for a short term—one to two weeks—to help us with a 'surgical camp' when we bring in thirty-five or forty children—typically with cleft lip and palate—for surgery. The most common volunteers are part of a surgical team that consists of surgeons, anesthesiologists, and nurses. We arrange for patients to come to the hospital for an intensive camp where we will perform thirty to forty surgeries in one week." The year-round operation of such a hospital staffed by surgeons means that there is capacity for follow-up after the volunteer camps by the permanent medical staff.

The CURE hospital in Niamey hosts about three surgical teams each year for seven to ten days, as well as some individual volunteers from the United States and Europe who stay for two weeks to a month. Lehman explains, "We also have volunteers that come to provide training; we work hard to be certain our clinical staff is meeting our high standard of care. The training volunteers typically spend time observing our staff, working with them one-on-one as they deliver patient care, and providing some lectures/classroom instruction on specific topics such as life support, medical math, protocols for certain types of procedures, or infection control."

CURE offers a good illustration of the role volunteers might play in one location where the services they offer are supplementary training and surgical interventions in a year-round facility. They add to what the hospital normally provides children by offering occasional intense weeks of specialized surgery, and they build additional capability by training the permanent staff. And since Niger is not on the itinerary of many sponsoring organizations, the hospital employees are especially appreciative of the volunteers who do come there.

On the other side of the globe is Heart to Heart International, which most commonly provides emergency assistance in response to disasters around the world. But in Haiti it has established a year-round operation. Haitian staffers, many of them employed directly by HHI, provide primary care services year-round in urban and rural clinics and are supplemented by regularly arriving volunteers.

Partnering with a church-based clinic in the capital, a pastor in a rural community, and regional peasant associations, HHI supports several clinics in different parts of the country. In the capital, the clinic is open most days of the week; outside the capital, clinics are held weekly or less often in churches or schools. Volunteers, including health professionals from around the United States, arrive frequently to stay for a week or occasionally a month. Among them are nurses from Bayada Home Health Care, a company headquartered in New Jersey, who receive time off from their employer to work in HHI clinics in Haiti. The visiting healthcare professionals provide skills and services similar to those provided by the Haitian medical staff, but their additional numbers make it possible to see more patients. Volunteers without medical training may assist in constructing facilities for visitors or providing community health education.

Each of these four different approaches to short-term volunteering can contribute, and each has potential disadvantages. But the fourth model—year-round operations with frequent short-term volunteers providing support for local professionals—is most likely to meet the criteria for excellent trips I discuss in later chapters. These include bringing needed skills and resources that are not available in the host community. Contributing skilled support to existing clinics, hospitals, and public health programs allows for continuity and predictability. Patients know when and where they can get help and that ideally their conditions can be followed up and side effects addressed.

Where They Go: Top Destinations

I asked what countries these organizations send their volunteers to, and 162 respondents listed specific countries (others mentioned continents or just said there were "many"). The top ten were Haiti (47), Honduras (32), India (31), Kenya (28), Uganda (24), Ecuador (23), Peru (21), Dominican Republic (20), Ghana (20), and Nicaragua (19).[3]

Most organizations send volunteers to more than one country—4.6 on average. When they send to only one, it is most frequently to Haiti,

India, Guatemala, or Cameroon. In all, organizations mentioned some 137 countries or territories, with 29 percent sending volunteers to list-leading Haiti. By far the most popular regions are Latin America and the Caribbean (two-thirds of organizations have at least one project in that region) and sub-Saharan Africa (somewhat under half have programs there). Few organizations work in the predominantly Arab countries of Western Asia and North Africa or in the countries of East and Central Asia, even fewer than those that place volunteers in the more developed countries of Europe and North America.[4]

Clearly there is an emphasis on poorer countries, but many destination countries are neither the poorest in the world nor the ones with the greatest levels of inequality and need, as measured by World Bank data.[5] Why these countries? I looked at a variety of factors—regional distribution, economic standing, and income inequality—but none of these entirely explains why organizations send volunteers to specific places.

Sending organizations take several key considerations into account when choosing destinations. For example, English is one of the official languages in India, Kenya, and Ghana, making it easier for American volunteers. Another important consideration is the need for stable organizational or individual partners who can sustain programs year-round and assist with arrangements and supervision. Ease of travel to the country is another important consideration, and that likely explains the dominance of Central and Latin American destinations for North American volunteers.

Safety is also a factor. For example, World Bank data suggest that Colombia has a higher level of inequality and presumably greater need than neighboring Ecuador, yet only two organizations send volunteers to Colombia, while twenty-three send them to Ecuador. This discrepancy is probably explained by the perception of greater danger in Colombia. By contrast, Haiti is by far the most frequently selected destination, even though the U.S. Department of State considers it unsafe. Its popularity is most likely due to a combination of other important considerations—a relatively short and inexpensive flight from the United States, a large population of Haitian Americans in the United States, its status as the poorest country in the Western Hemisphere, and, of course, the cataclysm that was the 2010 earthquake. Although many organizations worked in Haiti for only a few months after the earthquake, others introduced longer-lasting programs or continued programs that were in operation before 2010.

More often than not, the choice of destination results from individual preferences on the part of organizational founders, from relationships established with country nationals who have studied or visited in the United States, or though kin and community relations between people in the receiving countries and people living in the United States. Combinations of chance encounters and personal history are fairly typical in the history of volunteer-sending organizations.[6]

Timmy Global Health offers a case in point.[7] Matt MacGregor, Timmy's former executive director, explained to me how the organization began its work in Ecuador.

> Dr. Chuck had a relationship with a cancer patient here in Indianapolis who was half Ecuadorean. Chuck made what he would call a promise; he was very inspired by this woman, Margie Luna, who was the patient. Because of that he said, "Well, Margie, don't worry, I'm going to work in Ecuador. I'm going to work with your communities." And then when she passed away, he started actively working to create a project in Ecuador, so it was very much a product of an organic relationship that he met Padre Carollo [founder of the Tierra Nueva Foundation in Quito, which is one of Timmy's main partners for both outreach and referrals to the foundation's hospital] and then it started a relationship, which luckily has existed until today; I mean, it has thrived.

From this first start in Ecuador, Timmy Global Health sought projects in other countries as well.

> The same is true with our partnership in Guatemala that started in 2004; it was very much the product of a relationship developed by a student who was at that time an undergrad, then a med student who now is a doctor and still very involved with our programming and local partner organization. Since then, however, most of the other partnerships have been selected based on a more standardized metric. So for example, the Amazon Basin [in Ecuador] was selected because we wanted to work in a place that had 15 characteristics, including safety, ease of travel, significant need, strong local partner organization, existing local infrastructure and support systems, and a place that has significant need related to health. We have a lot of different

universities that want to work with us, and we need to pick a place that fits all these characteristics.

In many cases, volunteers' destinations are chosen individually rather than by an organization. People who want to volunteer may look for a volunteer matching organization that connects them to a specific country, or they may make their own arrangements. Students may find internship opportunities by connecting to a faculty member's project or through other personal contacts.

Dr. Giang Nguyen of the University of Pennsylvania School of Public Health, for example, works with students wanting global health internships but expects them to find their own placement. "Some of our students are immigrants themselves or come from immigrant families," he explains, "and they have some connections in other countries and they build on those. Others might work with organizations. They might have worked in public health locally with organizations that might have some connections elsewhere and some of them go that way, too."

The recruitment of immigrants in the United States for programs in their home countries can be seen in organized programs as well. For example, the Syrian American Medical Society has sponsored short-term medical trips to refugee camps in Turkey to provide primary care services to Syrians who have left their homes as a result of the civil war. Since the medical professionals are all Syrian in origin, they have the obvious advantage of being able to speak to and relate with patients.[8]

Average Length of Stay and Cost

The length of time volunteers stay in countries varies by organization and program. The same organization may sponsor a variety of programs of different lengths. For example, the great majority of Timmy Global Health's volunteers spend one week in country, but there are also a small number of longer-term volunteers who may stay for several months and work on special projects. Project Peru, which is based in Miami and sends medical volunteers to a clinic in rural Peru, organizes teams of medical professionals who stay for about ten days at a time, but the clinic also hosts medical and premed students for one to two months. A hospital director in Niger reported that volunteers there spend anywhere between two weeks and one year.

The most common length of time selected by organizers was two to three weeks, followed by a week or less. This confirms that the organizations focus almost entirely on very short-term volunteer activities.[9] Educational institutions are significantly more likely than faith-based organizations and NGOs to send volunteers for two to three weeks and significantly less likely to send them for a week or less.

With regard to cost, 35 percent of organizations report charging between $1,000 and $2,000 per volunteer. While almost one in ten agencies charges nothing, about 28 percent charge more than $2,000. Of those that do charge, the amount is generally a program fee and does not include airfare. Volunteers with faith-based organizations pay the highest, NGO volunteers pay the least, and educational institutions lie in between. This may be related to the length of the trip or the destination, but there is no obvious difference in these factors by type of organization, except that educational institutions send people for longer periods.

The U.S.-based organizations in my study sponsor an estimated 20,637 volunteers annually at an approximate average cost of about $1,500 per person, or an aggregate of at least $31 million per year (usually in addition to airfare). In the Catholic Health Association study, organizers estimated that nearly half of the total cost of medical missions goes for airfare. An important finding is that at best a quarter out of each dollar spent goes to the host country.[10]

Challenges to Program Effectiveness

I asked the representatives of volunteer-sponsoring organizations about the greatest challenges they face in sponsoring volunteer trips; they mentioned three most frequently: funding, coordination of effort during the trips, and managing expectations of volunteers and hosts. Also cited, but less frequently, were concerns about cultural barriers, sustainability, security, evaluation of impact, volunteer recruitment and commitment, and spiritual readiness. It becomes clear that the challenges are many.

Meeting the widely varying needs of volunteers, staff, and community members during an encounter across cultures, languages, and living conditions requires a lot of money to do well, so it is not surprising that funding was a top challenge cited. Money must be raised from donors and volunteers, and it must be available to pay overseas salaries when these are included. Additional funds for equipment and supplies and for unexpected emergencies must also be available.

The bottom line is that even with the best preparation, trips may not work out as planned. Bad weather, poor road conditions, battles over elections or territory, departure of key personnel, delays of medications in customs, last-minute volunteer cancellations—there are many conditions that may unexpectedly require a change in plans.

Hence the frequent reference to the challenges of coordination. "Logistics," it turns out, takes up a lot of organizers' time and effort. It is key to the success of international missions and can be quite challenging. Planning an international volunteer trip requires coordinating many individuals and groups at different levels of activity and expertise in at least two countries and involves myriad details. Organizers must recruit and select the right number of volunteers with needed expertise who are available on the projected dates. There are flights to reserve, transportation in country, and lodging and meals to arrange. Host-country rules, when they exist, about staff credentials and importing medications must be followed. Inexperienced volunteers must learn about shots and malaria medication and travel demands specific to their trip. Some organizations ask volunteers to bring extra supplies in their luggage in addition to the supplies and medication that are shipped or carried in by the organizers. All of this requires extensive coordination.

Then there are the many details regarding the actual program itself, including coordination with local partners and staff members and recruitment of patients when the program is not one that is continuous throughout the year. On top of that are all the unanticipated problems. Roads that under normal circumstances are barely passable may disappear altogether after heavy rains. Political changes at the national or regional level may lead to sudden changes in the personnel who were the expected partners, or worse, cause security concerns that lead to canceling a trip or ending it early.

Climate and technical problems can often pose challenges. One volunteer described to me how the generator in the hospital where they were carrying out training ran out of fuel. "We had no power, we had no air conditioner, we had no fan, and it had to be over one hundred degrees in there, and I just said, 'I'm really sorry. I'm going to try to make this as fast as I can.'" Sometimes, individual volunteers must be evacuated early because of illness or accidents.

Perhaps it is no wonder, given such difficulties, that "achieving sustainability" and "transcending cultural barriers"—both crucial dimensions of effective projects—were ranked close to the bottom of the list of challenges from which participants could choose. Cultural barriers include language and communication. "Two of the big problems we face are translators appropriately communicating with patients," says Matt MacGregor of Timmy Global Health, "and are our patients aware well in advance of when we're going to return and is that information distributed, because our whole continuity of care falls apart if our patients don't know when we're going to show up."

Evaluating impact was also not among the top challenges selected, and again we can see how it can easily take a back seat to the more immediate concerns. When asked about evaluation, an organizer I spoke with for the study carried out with the Catholic Health Association responded, "We have our own definition of success. We think, 'Well, that went well. You know, there were no major hiccups or disasters, so that went well!' Then we don't take the time to evaluate for improvement. That's an important thing that's often overlooked."[11]

In this hectic, shifting, challenging environment, intensified by the brevity of many trips, it is hard to pay attention to additional changes that might improve programs. But good organizations are the ones that are looking to evaluate what they do and to be sure that the programs they are involved in are having an impact.

Organizational Goals

In introducing the types of organizations that sponsor short-term health-related volunteering, I began to explore some of the organizational goals and motivations. Here I go into more specific detail about what sending organizations identify as their goals in sponsoring volunteers.

I asked organizers, "What do you consider your organization's or office's major goals with regard to global health?" The most frequent answers fall into a few categories: improving access to primary care, and a less-specific overall desire to improve health are the top two; just under a third of respondents offered one or both of these goals. Slightly more than 20 percent identified capacity building and missionary work as major goals. Other goals included improving access to specialty care, health education, providing good experiences for students and volunteers, research and training, disease prevention (including vaccination and nutrition), building partnerships, and improving water and sanitation.

Shift to other kinds of questions, though, and the focus on health services diminishes. Asked close-ended questions about other possible goals "that volunteers and/or internship programs help to achieve," half or more of the surveyed organizations agreed with the goals of fostering relationships with international partners, educating volunteers and interns, fund-raising, recruiting members or students, and enhancing the organization's reputation.

In follow-up interviews, most striking was the focus on goals other than health improvements. Three goal categories emerged as primary for the sponsors: providing health services and capacity building, enhancing the organization's reputation, and promoting volunteers' personal growth. Contributing to health is what we would expect as the main goal. But the other two are often considered just as important, raising questions about whether a focus on them might reduce the effectiveness of a group in promoting health.

Providing Health Services and Capacity Building   Providing direct health services is the most frequent type of activity of volunteer trips. Many of them also consider "capacity building," usually in the form of training of local personnel, to be a priority. A representative of an organization that had worked in Haiti in the immediate aftermath of the 2010 earthquake talked about how their goals had evolved over time, "[The first goal] was just fill the plane with people, get them down there to help, and that's how it started. . . . Treat the victims, because there were still so many victims. . . . The goal [now] is that this hospital will be run by Haitians and that we will be there more in a teaching capacity. . . . The goal that we're working towards [now] is a self-sufficient hospital that is run by Haitian staff. We'll be there as a tool."

A representative of FAVACA (Florida Association for Volunteer Action in the Caribbean and the Americas) an organization that matches consultants with specific projects, told me, "Our main mission is to improve the social and economic conditions in the Caribbean and the Americas. . . . We want to make sure that we're imparting knowledge; this is not just doctors seeing patients waiting in a long line, maybe giving them an aspirin or an antibiotic and then they leave next week. We always emphasize there has to be some system of training aspect to the project that you're leaving and imparting something to the partner, leaving it behind."

John Adams of PINCC in India emphasized the importance of training local healthcare workers to do some of his organization's work between visits. "If we just sent out teams to do the screening and treating, it wouldn't make a bit of difference in terms of the magnitude in the Third World; but if we train local healthcare workers to do the work and to train others to do the work, then the capacity building makes some sense. What we're trying to do is build up enough critical mass to pressure the government into getting involved."

Dr. Marjorie Muecke, assistant dean for Global Health Affairs at the University of Pennsylvania School of Nursing at the time of our interview, spoke of sending nursing students overseas and emphasized another dimension of capacity building: "What we care about is enhancing the work environment abroad for nursing so that nurses will want to stay in their own countries instead of leaving home to find better working conditions elsewhere."

In each instance, building some sort of health-related infrastructure and capability underlies the organization's efforts. For many other organizations, the goal is to provide primary care or surgical services to populations that lack adequate medical care. A typical comment came from the volunteer director of one sponsor organization: "The goal is to improve the healthcare access that people have in developing nations, most specifically within the communities that we're working on." Another stated a common goal of surgical volunteer programs: "They're very focused on delivering very high-quality surgeries, very quickly, so that in many people's mind, I can treat x number of people during this time period and I can do it very effectively."

Building Reputations   Organizations often sponsor volunteers in part to advance their own reputations, recruitment and retention efforts, or financial status. Educational institutions in particular need such programs to meet the demands of potential students. The director of study-abroad programs at a major state university remarked, "It's an important reputational thing; there's tremendous faculty interest in doing international work and research and so forth. The people in many leadership roles are very concerned about the reputational aspect, and is this something that will help us draw in more money."

Dr. Nguyen added that the reputational aspect is not only about fund-raising and student recruitment but also about international standing. "Of course we hope that when we send students, they're ambassadors for our university, they're ambassadors for our program."

Reputation and recruitment are also very important to corporations, and as corporate social responsibility becomes a more prevalent feature of the business world, global health volunteering helps promote a company's reputation—often in the face of bad publicity about corporate practices such as excessive profits or environmental damage. In some cases, corporate volunteering helps ease a company's entry into new markets.[12] Volunteer programs are also recognized as desirable to employees, many of whom value public service and want to see their employers involved.

One corporate director of social investing explained how volunteer activities contribute to employee recruitment and retention. "It really is helping to boost morale for associates, so that is definitely one of the purposes of the program. Yes, it is helping the community externally but then also inspiring the associates as well. The kind of person that the company wants to recruit is somebody who's very sensitive to public health, who wants to give back as part of a community approach. When we have university recruitment activities, we don't have the usual giveaways or pens or something like that but we're promoting one of our partners' activities to draw in students to learn more about us. It's OK to say that you want your associates to come back and be reinvigorated and inspired and have them think differently and to have a different perspective in their role."

Financial goals drive some volunteer recruiting as well. Volunteer fees are required if for-profit organizations are to turn a profit. This translates into little incentive to limit or screen volunteers, since more people means more money. I heard occasional stories of come-ons aimed more at generating income than good service: volunteers connected to projects by organizations driven by profit, with very little oversight and often very disappointing results for the volunteer.[13]

The motivation to have as many volunteers as possible also applies to nonprofits, for which volunteer fees comprise an important part of the budget for supporting their programs in host countries. These organizations recognize that volunteers who are impressed by the organization's work may become long-term donors and fund-raisers. I learned this lesson from a number of conversations, but one struck me as especially troubling. A man who had formerly worked in an organization that sends many young volunteers overseas told me that the organization's staff members were fully aware that volunteers were not accomplishing much when they went to poor countries. But they did not tell them this since their value was in later becoming sponsors to support the organization's work.

As mentioned earlier, building religious faith and church communities in other countries is a prevalent goal and could be considered part of enhancing the sponsoring institution. "As a Christian organization," one respondent wrote, "sharing our purpose and message of salvation in Jesus is our major goal." This goal pervades many faith-based medical trips.

But the benefits accrue to the sponsoring church as well. The sociologist Robert Wuthnow explains, "The church committees that organize these excursions anticipate larger gains as well. Seeing a mission station, school, or orphanage firsthand, they hope, will encourage church members to give more generously of their time and money in the future."[14]

Promoting Volunteers' Personal Growth   Many organizations emphasize the value volunteering has for the people who participate; for some, this is the primary goal. "For students who have not had international experiences or global health experience in general," says Dr. Nguyen, "I think that this gives them a sense of whether this is something they want to see as their career. It sounds exotic and everything and it's very exciting. I think that helps them understand what it really takes. So that's one of the major goals, just to give them real life experience in doing this so that they can decide for their future what they want to do."

Some people believe that sending medical residents to other countries can help educate them in the skills of cultural competency they will need as practitioners at home.[15] "The university's commitment is to help our students, our faculty and our staff to think like global citizens and become globally engaged in constructive ways," says Professor Muecke. Acknowledging that students are unlikely to make much of a difference for the host country, she adds, "I want the students in our short-term study-abroad courses to be transformed by the experience, even as short as most country field trips are."

For Steve Hower of Heart to Heart International, giving people the chance to serve is a primary consideration. "Our founder wants people to have an opportunity to serve; everybody has something to give and we want to find out what it is and help them find an opportunity to connect. It is about a transformation not only for the people who live here [in Haiti] but for the volunteer."

"Some [volunteer organizations]," adds Dr. Mark Rosenberg, CEO of the Task Force for Global Health, "are set up to bring volunteers to places for a short period of time to let the volunteers see what the real world is like and to give them an exciting exposure that doesn't focus on museums and gift shops but focuses on poor people and how they live."

Organizations sometimes consider an overseas trip a way to build leadership skills among employees, whether they work for hospitals or corporations. Several sponsors referred to the goal of using volunteer programs as a "stepping-stone or as a development program for leadership," in the words of one.

The volunteer experience may not be perceived by everyone as having such lofty goals as gaining cultural competence or education about other countries or even leadership development. Indeed, many organizations advertise for prospective volunteers by promising excitement and résumé building as the primary attractions.

I met with a premed student who wanted my help getting funding for a one-week medical trip to a Caribbean country. When I asked him why he wanted to go on the trip, he said, "There are so many rules in the U.S. about how much contact I can have with patients when I am shadowing doctors. I can do much more in another country." He added somewhat sheepishly, "And it will, of course, look very good on my medical school application."

I referred him to the literature on the ethical problems with premed volunteering overseas. But he may be correct about the advantages such a trip will give him. And many organizations see serving the personal goals of volunteers as an important part of their mission as well as a means of recruitment.

Most organizations have several goals they seek to achieve, and they often speak in terms of fulfilling two or three main goals at once. Timmy Global Health, for instance, "has a hybrid mission," explained Matt MacGregor. "Half of that mission is expanding access to health care. The other half of it—and I treat these goals almost equally—is very much about getting students and volunteers engaged in a responsible manner in global health activities. The explicit goal is to have them involved in work related to health disparities, global health, and health equity for the remainder of their career or their life."

Gregory Hodgson, the director of global health programs for Centura Health, outlines three primary goals in organizing overseas volunteer trips. "One is just the humanitarian goal of providing opportunities for people to seek care who otherwise wouldn't have access to that in developing countries. [T]hrough the [Catholic and Adventist] heritage that these hospitals have, they also have the goal of building capacity at mission hospitals supported by these religious organizations. [W]e also want to give our physicians and employees the opportunity to have the experience where they're working in a developing country as part of what we call our mission in ministry outside but also inside to our own employees and physicians. We feel that's an important experience that people can have."

Understanding organizations' goals in sponsoring short-term volunteer trips raises the question of whether meeting goals other than those focused on improving health may compete with meeting the needs of host communities. A primary goal of recruiting and educating students, for example, could result in sending unskilled and unprepared volunteers into a situation in which they may do harm or cost host communities time and difficulties without providing any benefit. Matthew Hunt and Beatrice Godard, who teach health professions students in Montreal, express concern about this conflict, particularly when students are seeking to gain research experience in poorer countries. The focus on student learning, combined with the students' lack of prior research experience, they write, "can limit the potential for . . . projects to be designed and implemented in ways that optimally address the health needs of local communities."[16]

Such conflicts exist in other types of volunteer trips. A primary goal of converting non-Christians could result in denigrating the beliefs of others or even excluding some people from services. And if increased morale among employees is a high priority, as in many corporate programs, there may be less attention to the actual value of what they do for host communities and more investment in the public relations aspects of their volunteering. For example, two of the dozen volunteers on the trip I accompanied to Haiti were there strictly for the purpose of creating PR materials.

In short, organizations that sponsor short-term health service trips often see important benefits to their own reputation, financial well-being, and recruitment potential; many goals for short-term volunteer activities identified by organizations have nothing to do specifically with improving health outcomes for people in the host communities. Of course, such trips can be valuable in improving health even when that is not their only purpose. But when goals conflict in ways that lead health improvements to be relegated to lesser importance or distorted by the other priorities, we need to be concerned.[17] And when poor and ill people are used as a vehicle for developing leaders for American organizations or career paths for privileged students or to diminish bad publicity for wealthy corporations, then we must raise the red flags to warn of exploitation and question the basic premise of this undertaking.

Part II

THE VOLUNTEERS

Who are the volunteers that travel overseas for a week or two or three to work with organizations providing health care, and why do they participate in these programs? Knowing more about these volunteers and what motivates them helps us understand what they bring to host communities.

We also look at how they are recruited, selected, and prepared. Many organizations accept almost anyone who volunteers, regardless of why the person wants to participate and whether or not he or she has any useful skills, while others are highly selective. Most organizations provide minimal preparation in advance of volunteer trips. When volunteers are not well screened and prepared, they face challenges in adapting to the work and the country that often diminish their potential contributions. Staff members who regularly work with volunteers in their own countries give us insights into how these volunteers might be better prepared before they arrive.

Many organizers, as well as many who write about volunteering, focus on the benefits to volunteers as an important goal of programs, as we saw earlier. Here we look at the evidence for those benefits and also some possible negatives. It becomes clear that there are ways to increase the positive impact on volunteers; these activities may also enhance the benefit to host communities.

3

BECOMING A VOLUNTEER

They have to have a passion to serve the Lord. . . . They have to be able to
sleep on the floor and work long hours.

Virtually everyone who can pay the fee is accepted.

— PARTICIPANTS IN SURVEY OF SPONSORING ORGANIZATIONS

Volunteer Recruitment and Selection

Considering the large number of organizations that are looking for volunteers, it is important to understand how they recruit them and how they screen them to be sure they are good candidates for a particular trip. When it comes to recruitment, an organization's Internet presence—its own website and social media—is by far the most important tool for recruiting volunteers, used by 62 percent of organizations. Word of mouth and targeted advertising through speaking engagements and letters are both second in importance. Hospitals, medical schools, universities, and churches recruit primarily from their own students, staff members, and congregants. Although more than half of the organizations describe themselves as faith-based, most of these recruit from other sources and not only from church organizations.

The Internet is also widely used by organizations in host countries to seek donors and volunteers from wealthier countries. Breezie Mitchell, an

American public health coordinator at a school in Kenya, describes how it works there. "Volunteers come to my site because the donors [in Europe] have put my organization on websites for people looking to volunteer for no cost. They offer free accommodations, so all that the volunteers have to pay for are travel and food expenses. The donors also have a website and blog, so anyone interested in volunteer experiences finds information about my organization that way."

Many organizations operate as conduits between volunteers and programs in other countries. For example, the medical director of a hospital in Niger reported, "We get our volunteers from three sources: SIM [Sudan Interior Mission]; Samaritan's Purse; and Medical Teams International [MTI]. The first two are Christian organizations and will only send us Christians; on the application there are questions about faith and beliefs. MTI, however, might send non-Christians but will only send experienced, well-qualified medical personnel, not students."

Prospective volunteers must typically follow some kind of written application process. Many organizations also use interviews and/or reference checks. "We screen every volunteer first by application review, then by phone interview," one participant explained. "If we feel confident after that, they may be chosen for a team. If we are not comfortable at that point, we will check references, or directly reject their application."

Another said, "They are interviewed by members of our medical committee who are in the same specialty. We require three references so those are also checked."

Others explained that the sponsoring church or club was responsible for screening or that screening would take place at an informal meeting followed by an interview. "We include someone from their church who knows them," wrote a representative of a faith-based organization, "and share the responsibility with them to decide if they are ready to go and going to do something that fits their skills and gifts."

Only a small number of organizations are highly selective. The majority accept almost anyone who applies; more than half of the organizations checked the option "76–100%" regarding the proportion of applicants they accept, with an additional one-quarter indicating they accepted between 51 and 75 percent. Indeed, 6 percent of the participants in our survey and 9 percent in the CHA survey do not screen volunteers at all.[1] "Virtually everyone who can pay the fee is accepted," wrote one participant. Another wrote, "We accept any one willing to come and work with us; we do not have any procedure."

Asked about specific skills or qualifications sought when recruiting, most organizations (60%) indicated general medical skills, including students in health profession schools. Next most important (25%) was some character trait such as flexibility or compassion. Specialized medical skills and other skills such as in business, law, construction, or public health were required by nearly a quarter of the organizations. Other qualifications cited less frequently were communication/language skills, being Christian, being able-bodied, and cultural sensitivity. "They have to have a passion to serve the Lord," wrote one respondent. "They have to be able to sleep on the floor and work long hours; they have to be able to withstand very hot weather."[2]

Fifteen percent of organizations indicated they require no specific skills. Minister Mable Humphrey, whose mission trips were described in chapter 2, represents the view of many sending organizations that do not require any specific skills. "Everyone has gifts," she said, "and I inspire and teach them to use their gifts. But people have to be obedient to the team." Since the team has many nonmedical activities (Bible teaching and prayer services, orphanage visiting, and educational projects) and also requires logistical support for the medical work, every volunteer can keep very busy during the trip.

My interviews also revealed a wide range of criteria for selecting volunteers. For example, Sandy Del Prado, founder of the Kausay Wasi Clinic in Coya, Peru (part of Project Peru), requires specific medical and linguistic skills. "Doctors and nurses *must* be experienced. As to students, we prefer offering the opportunity to premed or medical students who seek a career in the health field. Conversational Spanish is required for students, who also serve as interpreters for visiting medical teams. We also prefer students with a history of volunteer activities."

Although most organizations have criteria for accepting or rejecting applicants, they often leave the decision up to a team leader (e.g., college chapter officer or church group leader). In many cases, volunteers are spread throughout the United States, and there may not be an opportunity for an in-person encounter. Credential checks are employed primarily for medical personnel who will be practicing medicine in the host country; organizations may then do a background check for licensing, malpractice history, and so on. But when an organization expresses a preference for a person with particular personal qualities—someone who is adaptable or compassionate, for example—it is impossible to know in advance whether a volunteer applicant has those desired attributes.

The fact that organizations include so many people with limited skills and experience raises critical questions about the quality of medical care that they can provide. But remember that for many organizations, providing care is only part of their mission. Those who also believe it is important to give Americans an exposure to other cultures and to poverty and those who use volunteer fees to fund their organizations are motivated to include as many volunteers as possible. They find tasks for them to do, such as loading and unloading supplies, taking vital signs, or painting and repairing buildings.

Of course, these are activities that could be done more inexpensively and with greater benefit to local communities if the residents of those communities were hired to do them. Many volunteers come away from their experiences with a vague sense of dissatisfaction at not having been able to do much that was useful. In fact "managing volunteer expectations" was cited as a leading challenge by organizers of international medical missions.[3]

Lack of selectivity can have a number of negative consequences. It privileges the acquisition of experience by well-off Americans over the needs of poorer host communities. It can waste the time and resources of organizers and hosts who have to deal with unskilled and occasionally uncooperative or disruptive visitors. It can undermine work opportunities for host community members. And it can mean a dissatisfying experience for the volunteer whose expectations for contributing something are not met.

I wondered what would lead an organization to reject an applicant. Organizers most frequently cited poor adaptability, believing the applicant could not work as part of a team or had a poor attitude. Other reasons include theological incompatibility (obviously applying to some faith-based groups), inadequate skills (including low grades in school, poor communication, and poor or no language skills), poor recommendations, criminal history, malpractice, health issues, or noncompliance with rules or paperwork. In some cases, an applicant is rejected because there is insufficient space on a specific trip or because he or she will not be available when needed.

Some representatives of organizations who seek experienced medical professionals told me they face the challenge that some medical personnel have a difficult time adapting to the work conditions they will face or to the requirement of working in a team that they are not in charge of. Hence the concern by many organizers to find people with the personality and interpersonal qualities needed for the situation.

The fact that some organizations take anyone who applies and can pay the fee comports with the philosophy of people such as Dr. Gary Morsch of Heart to Heart International who believe everyone has something to contribute and that the organization can find a way to make that happen.[4] It may also, in some cases, reflect a certain recklessness and/or profit motive with the potential to backfire once a volunteer is in the field.

Researchers in 2005 found many examples of programs they considered "shallow" and lacking impact, and one of the key characteristics in their analysis is volunteers' lack of skills. For example, they cite a 2003 announcement from Cross-Cultural Solutions that describes "volunteer work on sustainable community development projects with infants and children, teenagers, adults, the elderly and people with special needs like HIV/AIDS patients, or the mentally or physically disabled." Notably, volunteers need not have any skills or experience to participate. They also indicate that of 295 "community welfare" projects identified, only 24 percent required the volunteer speak the local language.[5]

Their examples are neither unusual nor outdated. More recently, in 2013, the organization Unite for Sight, which has eye-care programs in many countries and recruits heavily among students, sent out mass e-mails with this message: "We are excited to announce a new 1-week Ghana Volunteer Abroad Program opportunity! Select any Saturday-Saturday program dates during 2013 or 2014, and participate with Crystal Eye Clinic's extraordinary doctors to provide care for patients living in extreme poverty. . . . There is no formal application to participate in this new 1-week program, and you may simply enroll online. Those enrolling by June 30, during this first launch week, receive a $100 discount."

Unite for Sight also offers a "Global Impact Fellow" program, which places volunteers for several weeks or months in Honduras, India, and Ghana. This program, according to the website, is "suitable to anyone 18 years and older who has an interest in international service, global health, and social entrepreneurship."[6] The lack of any mention of screening at all is a concern. Yet an officer of Unite for Sight told me in a phone conversation that even the one-week volunteers have to write application essays and might be rejected, while the Global Impact Fellows must submit letters of recommendation as well.

At least Unite for Sight has an online course that volunteers must pass before they travel. This is a much more in-depth preparation for the country and the details of eye care than most prospective volunteers receive.[7] Additionally, the volunteers are employed in ongoing clinic activities, usually providing initial eye screening or checking in patients. The wholesale recruitment of short-term volunteers is certainly an effective fund-raising mechanism, as the entire $1,800 program fee is directed at service provision. Volunteers are expected to raise funds or pay that amount, in addition to paying for airfare and living expenses in the countries they visit.

Different Approaches to Preparation

One would think that traveling to another country for something other than sightseeing would require significant preparation, especially if it involves considerable interaction with local people. Expecting a young and inexperienced person (a large proportion of the volunteers fit this description) or even a mature professional to arrive in an unfamiliar environment and begin to work productively for a week or two requires effective preparation beforehand and organization while on the ground.

So I asked sending organizations what type of information they provide volunteers before they leave and whether they have some kind of orientation. More than 90 percent do provide an information packet with advice about travel, shots, and packing. Nearly three-quarters include reading materials about the country to be visited. And more than half have an in-person orientation program, although many of these do not take place until the volunteer arrives in the country. About one in three offers an online orientation.

Simply sending materials to volunteers is no guarantee they will be studied. One organization I spoke with works primarily with college students and sends materials out prior to travel—and then *hopes* they're read. "What we really try to do is constantly reassess how the trip is set out for students prior to travel, what they're expecting to do, how they're expecting to spend their days, where they'll be living," I was told. "We really work to spell out exactly what they'll be doing. We very honestly have lines that say you are fully expected to read all of the materials that are presented to you prior to your travel, so we do what we can."

What comprises an orientation? In addition to practical information regarding travel, most organizations discuss the planning of activities that will be carried out, and over 70 percent indicated that the orientation provides "cultural competence for the specific country." Some history of the country is provided in just over half the orientations. However, my own observations and interviews with senders raise questions about whether cultural understanding and history preparation are anything more than superficial in many cases.

Organizations are much less likely to include the other elements of an orientation about which I asked. Slightly fewer than a third of them bring in staff members from the hosting country to meet with volunteers or provide any training in specific skills needed for the project. Nearly 10 percent provide no orientation whatsoever.

"Some volunteers arrive on site without any contextual understanding beyond what makes headlines," says Barrett Frankel, an American working with volunteers in Rwanda. "They don't realize that because something works in X location does not mean it will succeed in our village. They arrive and think they can 'fix' something, without giving any thought to whether that something is really broken as it exists."

The bottom line is that organizations vary greatly in their philosophies and practices regarding the preparation of volunteers. Some provide basic travel information and little more. Others have much more in-depth preparation; this is the case for educational institutions in particular, some of which offer credit-bearing courses in which service trips are embedded.

Dr. Nguyen tells students "to go to the CDC website, search out the place you're going to go, find out what's required and think about what are some of the major health issues that are affecting the country that you're going to, and also prepare yourself medically if necessary. See your own doctor and get your immunizations and get your malaria prophylaxis. And in cases where they are planning a particular project, then I of course would require that they do some literature review in advance so that they really know what is the state of knowledge concerning the topic."

These students, continues Dr. Nguyen, "most likely will have taken the Introduction to Global Health course and other core courses in public health—Introduction to Statistics, Introduction to Epidemiology, all those types of things required for all of our public health students."

An example of a more focused and unusual approach is the one adopted by the organization Amizade, whose goal in preparing the college students it works with is to foster a challenging and critical conversation about the context in which volunteering takes place. Brandon Blache-Cohen described the organization's approach. "We ask them to read a lot of pieces that are telling them that they *shouldn't* be going to Mexico, they *shouldn't* be working in Bolivia, they're hurting communities by doing this. Basically, they're asked to think of the stereotypes and what they think of these communities of service–what is service? That's a big thing, because students have this belief that service is hammer and nails. Ultimately what I think happens on a good program is that students start to reflect on how it is they can best make an impact on the world. [T]he pieces that the students are reading typically are going against everything they've been brought up with."

FAVACA adopts a very different strategy: rather than employing group brigades, it generally matches individual consultants who possess specific advanced skills with targeted projects. "We really prepare them," Chris Beyer told me at the South Florida office. [The volunteer and host organization] ask each other questions. E-mails are going back and forth. They know where they're going to stay. They know who's picking them up. The person will have such and such a hat on. We also hold orientation calls with many of our volunteers. We send them an orientation binder, which goes over our rules and policies, how best to conduct yourself abroad, and answers all sorts of questions individuals may have, especially if they have never traveled abroad, giving them travel tips, health tips, how to convert currency, how best to conduct yourself in a particular culture."

The faith-based hospital system Centura Health uses online videos and hopes to expand its Web-based preparations. "What I'm really working on trying to develop now," says Greg Hodgson, director of Global Services, "is where we have interactive Web-based programs where they can go through a little training module where they'd have a little quiz or something along the way making sure that they understand and don't have to sit through a one-hour lecture of something at the university."

Online preparation is not unique to Centura Health. The University of Minnesota, notes Tricia Todd, has developed a required online program for prehealth and health profession students going abroad. The "Global Ambassadors for Patient Safety" program emphasizes what students should and should not be doing in patient-care situations if they are untrained. As mentioned above, Unite for Sight requires that all volunteers complete a series of online modules before they depart.

Many organizations provide a brief orientation for volunteers once they arrive in the host country. The director of volunteers for an NGO that sends primarily students on short-term trips explains, "Usually they arrive in the afternoon or evening on a weekend. They'll be driven to their homestay, meet their homestay family, and the next morning they'll be picked up and they'll go to the clinic. First thing, they'll do an orientation to the clinic with the field operations manager, get the ground rules, get the plan for the week, and then they'll jump right in to whatever it is they're doing."

Often, orientation occurs in the host country just as the volunteers are beginning to work, with not even the limited time to acclimate described in the example above. "When they get to the hospital," the representative of an organization that sends primarily health professionals told me,

> the first thing they do is have an orientation. They get oriented to the hospital, to what the goal is, to what they'll be doing, and then half of them start working immediately, because what happens is we try to bring the group in in the morning and send the last group out at the last flight so they can hand it off. They can talk to the staff that's been there, find out about the patients, about what's been going on, and then one group leaves and the next one takes over. [The permanent hospital staff] gets the information before. They know who's coming and they pretty much kind of put it together and say, "Okay, here's the work. You're going to go there. You're going there. This is how you're going to work. You're working day, you're working nights."

The two trips I participated in, one through Timmy Global Health in Ecuador and the other sponsored by Becton Dickinson in partnership with Heart to Heart International in Haiti, both offered primary care in clinics. While they were quite different in their approach to volunteer orientation, neither provided much preparation for the countries and cultures to be encountered.

BD's orientation lasted for two and a half days and brought volunteers together from around the United States and several other countries a few months in advance of the planned trip. This was obviously a very expensive project that nonprofits would be hard-pressed to duplicate. It was an opportunity for the volunteers to meet each other, get their immunization shots, learn about the organization's goals, and plan the specific projects that they would be engaged in. However, information about the country and its culture and language comprised only about an hour of the total time we were together and was not especially informative. This in spite of the fact that my students who had accompanied earlier volunteer trips with BD in Ghana reported back to the company's leadership about the need for much more advanced training in cultural competence.

My trip to Ecuador included no advance orientation. Materials about travel, arrival at the airport, itinerary in the country, drinking water, and items to pack arrived by e-mail. Attention to the need for deeper reflection on the meaning of this upcoming encounter was summed up in a message from the American staff person we would soon meet: "Your week here in Ecuador will be an unbelievable opportunity to learn more about a developing country, witness poverty firsthand, practice your Spanish, and serve people in much need of your time, energy, and hope. It will also be a week to reflect on yourselves—your beliefs, attitudes, and life goals. As a former brigade volunteer, I can say without hesitation that your brigade week will be one of the most fun, challenging, and eye-opening experiences. But remember that the brigade only lasts a week, so come with an open mind, a flexible attitude, and a sense of humor."

When we arrived in Ecuador, there was a meeting in which we were introduced to how the tasks would be distributed during clinic days and each evening in preparation for the next day's clinics. We were given no information about the country, cultural issues, or language. At one clinic, a village official greeted us in Kichwa, the local language, but most of the volunteers did not recognize what he was saying and could not respond. Clearly an opportunity lost.

In contrast, in Pennsylvania I attended the first of several weekly sessions for members of a local church who were preparing a trip to Haiti. Several of the volunteers were Haitian Americans, and others had visited

Haiti before; they talked about the country and culture and what to expect. This orientation emphasized the evangelical mission of the trip. It began with a prayer and a Bible reading from Matthew 28:19–20: "Therefore go and make disciples of all nations, baptizing them in the name of the Father and of the Son and of the Holy Spirit, and teaching them to obey everything I have commanded you. And surely I am with you always, to the very end of the age." The leader, Minister Mable Humphrey, emphasized that their purpose was to show that the parishioners cared by bringing medicine and "establishing not only the body of Christ but establishing a medical facility and creating jobs." These injunctions were followed by very practical information about packing and advice on how the group should behave in various situations, such as in response to requests for gifts.

Whether this one trip, which was part of a series of occasional visits by the same American church group, would accomplish anything for the host community's health or create jobs was not clear to me when I was at the pretrip meeting. But the volunteers, because they live in the same region and many go to the same church, at least had the advantage of being able to coalesce into a working team and learn about Haiti before they arrived as well as address some of the obstacles they might experience—something I did not observe in other preparatory situations.

What Hosts Think Volunteers Should Know before They Arrive

When I asked host-country staff members what they would want volunteers to know about their communities or about the work they'd be doing *before* they arrived, the responses indicated their desire for volunteers to know quite a lot more about the country than they did. This included the country's history, its climate, and the health needs they would encounter.

One of the most frequently mentioned issues in every one of the four countries where we conducted interviews was that of language and culture. "It's always good to know the language wherever you're going," a Haitian staff member told me, "not only for work, but if I go to the States, I speak English and if I want to go to Mexico, it would be good to speak Spanish even though you don't speak it correctly. But the basic things; if you know them, that will be helpful." The lack of language skills among volunteers creates challenges. Another Haitian told me, "It's true that it's a little difficult because sometimes volunteers want to come, but they don't speak the language. So we have to have translators."

Host-country staff members want volunteers to know more about their cultures as well as their language. An Ecuadorian suggests volunteers should be given "a brief cultural background, a brief political background, and a brief economic background, because you need to understand the environment a little bit better. I've heard a couple times, for example, some people thought that Ecuador is a dictatorship, and it's kind of funny, but it's misinformation. I remember a student asking me if we know what a democracy is and if we live in a democracy. And I was thinking, 'Man, you didn't read anything about the country when you came, right?' The good thing is that he was interested to know. I'm sure if people could get more information before they came, it would be more rich for them."

For some host staff members, the important cultural information focused on religious practices. A hospital employee in Niger responded to the question of what volunteers should know by saying, "Depending on the month they come, it's a Muslim-majority country and there are things you don't do." This reference to Ramadan practices underscores that many customs taken for granted in other countries are unfamiliar to most Americans, and volunteers could easily cause offense without realizing it. The man continued, "I would give them advice on taking time to get to know people, to be ready to drop your preconceived ideas."

A few people responded to the question about what volunteers should know by focusing on safety issues. A staff member in Niger wanted outsiders to be cautious about possible violence in the north of the country; in contrast, a Haitian physician was concerned that foreigners would be overly worried about safety. "Some people, when they come into Haiti," he said, "think Haiti is a bad country, it's not really safe, and there's a lot of kidnapping, so we talk to them about that, let them know it's not really true. You know everywhere around the world there's problems, not only in Haiti."

Other host staff members would like volunteers to have a sense of the needs of the country and the work they'll be doing before they arrive. A Ghanaian specifically mentioned the socioeconomic conditions of the people. "I would begin by [talking about] work," said a host staff member in

Niger. "And what medical situations they are going to see on the ground." A colleague said, "First I'm going to show them that they are going to enter a country that is less rich than their own and it's possible that they are going to see a lack of materials with which to work, a lack of products."

The importance of having some advance knowledge of the specific health conditions is frequently cited. "I would take the opportunity to tell them about the kind of environment they're coming into," says a Ghanaian. "This hospital, for instance, the kind of inpatients we usually have, the kind of people they're going to come in contact with, maybe possible problems they'd face."

Barrett Frankel, an American who has received international volunteers at a youth center in Rwanda, answered the question about what volunteers should know with the following response, which incorporates several kinds of advice offered by others:

> I tell them during orientation that they should be diplomatic and somewhat cautious when entering into certain topics that include subject matters such as politics and religion. I remind them that they are going to be staying in rural Rwanda where electricity is at times scarce, the water often runs out, and the Internet is slow at best. Showers are cold, the sun is hot, and hand sanitizer should be their best friend. I remind them to have manners and not outwardly show their disapproval or disappointment about cultural norms or the lackluster food, as respect is highly coveted here. Modesty is essential. Lastly I would remind them that their stay is limited, so not to promise anything they cannot or will not deliver when it comes to the students.

As we've seen, most organizations provide very little advance preparation, and orientations are brief and often occur just as volunteers are launched into their work. Many of them do provide basic information about climate and what to pack, but it is much harder to prepare outsiders for language and cultural differences beyond the most superficial elements. Yet this is clearly an important gap identified by many of the staff members who receive volunteers, and it is part of the rationale for longer stays during which the volunteer may have more of an opportunity to learn about the country and adapt to the needs of the work environment.

Quito Airport, Ecuador, 2012. It is 1:00 a.m., and my student Joe and I are still waiting to get through passport control. I have way too much time to study the large Coca-Cola advertisement on the wall in Spanish, "Smile. Quito welcomes you." I do feel welcomed and eager to get started, although I wonder exactly what we'll be doing in the week to come.

After a full day of tourism, enjoyable despite lack of sleep and some altitude sickness, we are on a bus heading toward the Amazon Basin. Our home for the week reminds me of summer camp, with bunk buildings and a central dining room. After dinner, we gather in a large circle for our first formal orientation, forty Americans from a wide variety of backgrounds, ranging from ages twenty to seventy. They call us a brigade, but we don't yet know what that will mean.

Each of us is given an assignment to carry out every evening to prepare for the next day's clinic. Some bag and label pills, marking names and dosages. Others fill plastic bins with supplies. My job is to stock a suitcase with the materials for providing fluoride treatment to children, along with toys to attract them to hang out with the volunteer doing the treatments.

Evening is also when many volunteers head to a nearby bar. I'm sure some people aren't getting a lot of sleep. Yet we're all there for breakfast early each morning, where excited monkeys greet us around the edges of our dining pavilion. Some young men on our brigade jump up and down to scare the monkeys away. I wonder who looks sillier.

By 7:30 a.m. there is a rapid deployment of ready hands as supplies are loaded quickly onto our bus to the village. I'm impressed by the men who load three heavy bins at once. Some climb up on top of the bus to what looks like a very unsafe perch for the bumpy ride. There seems to be a great deal of testosterone flowing in our group.

Every day, the team goes to a different village and sets up a clinic in a central community building. Local community health workers have sold tickets for the clinic in advance, fifty cents apiece. Scores of patients and family members are already waiting when we arrive.

The community workers in a typical clinic set up three doctor stations on the stage, screened by blankets hanging from a line and separated by benches. Volunteers unload the bus and begin setting up intake and history, vitals, lab, and pharmacy stations at tables and benches scattered around the large room. The "lab" is a table staffed by a nurse with some supplies for urinalysis, pregnancy tests, and a few procedures. An area out back is designated for patients to go to fill their pee cups.

Once we are set up, patients who have gone through intake and had their vitals checked can see one of the volunteer doctors and then move through to the pharmacy for any prescribed medications. I get to observe and help out where I can. Patients tell of everyday aches from working in the fields and sometimes of injuries from accidents. Almost all, children included, suffer headaches or muscle aches. One doctor emphasizes drinking more water to avoid dehydration and thus reduce the headaches.

As soon as the symptoms start seeming routine, we meet a woman with advanced cancer. The doctor says that she cannot be helped, and the young, inexperienced translator has to convey the bad news. It is a tough day for the translator.

Outside, children are playing soccer with a volunteer and getting their teeth treated with fluoride. Some get antiparasite treatment. At the end of the day, we pack everything up, load it on the bus, and return to our base for showers, dinner, pill packing, and beer. It's been a long, satisfying, intense day. The volunteers have worked hard and forged a good team spirit, but we're clearly outsiders. We have minimal interaction with the Ecuadorean staff or patients.

The next brigade should be returning to the same village in about two months. Meanwhile, some patients will be accompanied to hospitals for more advanced care.

Volunteer Adaptation

Comments from organizational sponsors, volunteers, and hosts all suggest that some of the very brief work hours available to volunteers during their short visits may be lost because of the time they end up having to spend adapting to a situation for which they could have been better prepared. The challenges to new volunteers include adapting not just to the work but also to the country environment—everything from transportation to the weather.

Of course, no orientation can completely prepare volunteers for what they will experience in a new situation. Regardless of preparation, volunteers arriving in a country they have never visited will inevitably require some time to get used to the new environment. Since many visits are for only a week or two, the time for adapting is often insufficient. They are expected to begin working almost immediately in a situation very different from their norm. Fortunately, volunteers mostly do seem to manage to adapt fairly quickly to the environment and the needs of the work situation.

But this does require flexibility and the ability to respond to unexpected situations. A Haitian medical professional gave one example of how Americans may not understand the conditions local staff members often encounter: "If you are Haitian and you have to come to work at 8:00 and you live far away and you come at 8:30 or 9:00, it could be hard for an American to understand that. 'How come you're so late and blah, blah, blah, blah, blah?' Not only do they have to take three *tap taps* [local minibuses]; in Haiti today everything is fine but tomorrow you have barricades, you have, you know, many things. You can't really set up your time, say OK, from here to there is going to take me thirty minutes, like in the States."

Another Haitian mentions the roads. "It's not easy because sometimes people come and they're in Haiti for the first time. And you know how difficult the roads are in the south especially and it's very hard to adapt. But they often show that they're very interested and that they don't have a problem with traveling and they'll accept the conditions of travel, the living conditions, which are pretty different from those of the volunteers' house in the capital. There are some who don't adapt as well; they're all a bit different."

A volunteer in a rural part of Haiti concurs. "One of the priority problems we identified was road access. No one wants to go there. It was a rough ride! It's a very demanding ride, very, very demanding physically." This volunteer worked in a town that is about ninety-five miles from the capital in a beautiful mountain region. Because of the poor quality, or in many cases the total lack, of roads, the trip from the capital can take as much as eight hours. Another volunteer described the route as "bone-rattling."

Being prepared for the weather is key, too. "It's especially necessary to know what time [of year] they'll be coming," says a staff member in Niger, "because there's the cold season and the hot season. If they are used to heat, I want to tell them to come in that period; they should come. Look at how hot it is in the shade, in the sun, and compare that to where you're from. The most important thing when volunteers come here is health, housing, and security. Food is part of that."

The physical conditions can take a toll. When I was in Ecuador, a fair number of our group—including some of the experienced people—suffered from stomach ailments and diarrhea. One volunteer had to be admitted to a hospital because he was so ill and dehydrated. Fortunately, he was able to continue with the trip the next day, but it is not unusual for volunteers to suffer from illness or injury.

Even without illness, there are physical demands to which volunteers are not accustomed. In our group discussion our last night in Ecuador, one volunteer said, "I think I underestimated the kind of physical stamina that is necessary for this brigade. I think yesterday and the day before were particularly hard, and there were moments when I felt I was starting to get really, really dehydrated and stuff, so that's something I need to keep in mind for preparation for the future."

A volunteer in Haiti told his story on the last night during group discussion. "The other night we were trying to get everything ready for the next day. [One of the volunteers, an experienced nurse] goes to the bathroom, and all of a sudden you hear this great big scream: 'Oh, my god! It's a nightmare!' So I come running and there's about ten massive cockroaches in the bathroom, all over the tub, the walls. We're like, 'Oh, my god, we haven't had a shower yet.' So we had to kill them all before we could have a shower. We had to fumigate." We managed to have a good laugh over an experienced nurse freaking out about bugs.

Far worse than adapting to bugs and heat and cold showers, for medical professionals especially, is seeing patients suffer and die for lack of facilities and supplies. "Today was very emotional," a nurse volunteer recounted in a group meeting. "We had a baby that was really so badly anemic, I've never seen that before, and we brought the baby to the hospital in Leogane, and they were saying there was no blood in the place, only in Port-au-Prince, so they were not sure that this baby could be transfused. The mother was anemic, too, very badly. They were going to make tests for the father, but they were not sure it would be OK to transfuse the baby with the father's blood. In our countries, something like that is easy, I mean, we go to the hospital, there is a blood bank and we can fix this sort of thing easily, and here, the baby is there, but there is no blood, and we don't know if this little, two-month baby is going to survive, so it was really sort of emotional."

Adapting to the work also presents challenges. "There is a lot of eye opening in the first week," says the medical director of a hospital in Niger. "There is a steep learning curve." The fact that so many volunteers have not been specifically trained for the work they're going to do figures into the equation.

"I think a lot of it is training, too," says the representative of a sponsor organization. "I think we throw people into situations sometimes and don't explain things to them, don't teach them things."

Even skilled professionals require some time to become familiar with the place in which they'll be working, the available supplies, and the procedures to be followed. I have seen some volunteers adapt quickly and intelligently but often by coming up with their own procedures rather than having things clearly defined from the start. In both countries where I participated in and observed volunteer teams in primary care clinics, I noticed we were often figuring out procedures on our own at the beginning. For many volunteers, their own training and work experience are very different from what they are called on to do. Thus clinic procedures can have an ad hoc quality, which can change over the course of the time they spend, as volunteers gain more experience and greater confidence.

I noted in Haiti that the nurse volunteers had not been working as nurses back home; although trained in nursing, they had been doing other work for a number of years. One nurse's prior experience, already several years removed, had been in a neonatal intensive care unit, not in primary care. One said she had to figure out the different names of medications, which took a couple of days, before she was able to learn to explain dosage in Creole.

The lack of well-matched experience can be a serious issue. In Ecuador, I spoke with two of the volunteers, a physician and a nurse, who were both worried about a bad fit between their skills and the jobs that needed to be done. For example, the nurse hadn't practiced nursing for four years and was being called on to perform procedures she hadn't done for a while. She felt strongly that having a nursing license wasn't enough. The physician worried that she was not able to take a full history and couldn't get the information she needed. She felt most patients didn't need MDs to deal with the aches and pains that were among the most commonly presented symptoms and that patients with more serious problems could not be helped. Back home, she saved patients every day, she told me. In Ecuador, it was often too late to help a sick patient, or there was nothing available. Both felt they were not really saving lives and not doing good medicine. The physician had wanted to volunteer for years, but after two days she was feeling demoralized.

An American nurse volunteer in Haiti told me that on the first day the nurses had no idea what they were doing, where things were located and what was available, or what procedures to follow. They finally figured it out, but it took a while, and the interpreters had apparently not been empowered to guide them. They eventually fell into a pattern, and when there were two triage teams working side by side, one led by the nurse and the other by an EMT-trained volunteer, they listened in to each other's intake interviews to see how the other one asked questions and were able to learn from each other.

As I wrote in my field notes at the time, "It would be better if volunteers were better prepared or local staff such as translators had more authority to do some of the intake since they know what the questions are. Or if the medical volunteers had much more specific information about symptoms and follow-up questions and how to ask them. They did get a manual from the NGO before they came, but they did not think that was sufficient."

What I observed is quite common, both in primary care situations and in health education. One organization asks students with no teaching or health experience to do brief research and then present to local community members the health education lessons they have created. Even volunteers with more training and experience express concerns about having to figure out what to do. One community health trainer working for Heart to Heart International in Haiti told me, "There was a lack of protocols. You have to figure it out yourself. Some of the information I got from a great book I downloaded, *Where There Is No Doctor*. There is information from the World Health Organization that's used in developing countries that's basic—hygiene, sanitation-type information—so I downloaded a bunch of that stuff on my laptop and brought it here."

Figuring it out yourself hardly seems the way to run a health program, especially when every week or two another set of new people have to once again figure it out. Even when there is guidance from the local staff or program organizers, new volunteers are not very different from new employees, who require time to learn the ropes and find a way to perform their new tasks. It's as if every day in American hospitals were July 1, the day new, inexperienced residents arrive and when—as is widely believed—medical mistakes increase.

Health professionals can find it especially difficult to adapt to local conditions that are very different from what they are used to at home. "The doctor in charge sort of told us what to do," said a nurse volunteer, "but I don't think we really understood. It's hard with the two translators because one's doing crowd control for a good part of the time and then I thought, well, what am I supposed to be doing? And it's kind of going back to your nursing days to have to try and think of these things, so it was a good review to do things like that. But for the whole 'are you sexually active' thing—so out of my element."

A lack of supplies seemed to be a regular problem to which volunteers must adapt. As a volunteer nurse told me,

> We were missing some stuff most of the time, and sometimes simple stuff like Ziploc bags, like glasses to put the water in for the syrup for the kids or simple things like that. I had to make a lot of IM injections but I had almost no IM needles. I took the needles I had but I'm not sure the product was even in the muscle. Also, something to wash your hands for the staff, because if you want to wash your hands, you just can't and it's very dusty. Well, before injections I didn't feel really comfortable with that, even if we had the sanitizer and everything, but washing and sanitizing are not the same.

The challenge of providing effective services without understanding the local language is one of the issues often mentioned by host-country staff members, as we saw earlier. Volunteers also recognize the language barrier as a problem, and for many the biggest challenge of being in a different country is not being able to communicate. In a volunteer gathering my last evening in Ecuador, many expressed regrets about not speaking Spanish. "I can't speak a word of Spanish," said one volunteer, "and neither can I understand anything. I would have loved to talk to the people and get to know them better and know about their lives, their cultures."

"Any time you work through a translator," said another volunteer, "I think it's much more difficult to do education, and it's more difficult to make sure you're doing the education well." Working through interpreters also means taking a great deal more time to see a patient; surely the interpreters could do the intake more efficiently and accurately with some training.

During the group session on the last night in Haiti, a laboratory trainer recounted the challenges of teaching with interpreters. "It started off kind of shaky, at least for me, because it was my first time using a translator and a different language, making sure that what you said was the right message that got out. Our translators got better over the course of the week to the point where they know the material as much as we do, which was really, really awesome. The first day you kind of forget that the translator is supposed to be there, so then I would just start rambling, thinking that you should understand what I'm saying. So it's definitely different."

I also noticed other challenging communications problems. There was a striking lack of personal interaction with patients despite the volunteers' best efforts; of course, language is part of that. I also saw the difficulty in asking patients certain types of questions. When the nurse or paramedic doing intake asked how long a patient had had a symptom, some found it difficult to say, and the interpreter would, with some humor, chastise them for not answering the question and would repeat, "How many days, how many weeks, how many months, how many years?" As I wrote in my field notes, "There should be a better way to do this."

Once, a volunteer doing intake asked patients with vaginal infections whether they wore panties made of synthetic material. The interpreter, using the French word, asked whether their panties were "synthétique," which patients did not seem to understand. I suggested asking instead whether they were cotton, which seemed to work. It is difficult to see how these issues of communication would *not* figure into a calculation of whether host communities get value out of the volunteer visits.

The time factor exacerbates all the adaptation issues. The last night in Ecuador, one of the volunteers captured some of the drawbacks of brief volunteer missions. "I felt like today I've now tried pretty much every station in the brigade at least for a little bit, and I finally feel like I'm kind of getting the hang of it, so now I'm going to have to come back and do it all again." This may be good for the next time, if there is one, but it represents a very regrettable loss of time and effectiveness for a large part of the current trip.

Adapt, though, they must. "One of the key words that certainly my team learned is to adapt," a volunteer told me. "You can plan all you want, you can foresee all you want, but it won't go as planned, so that's one of the things that I'll take along."

4

What Leads to Volunteering, What Volunteering Leads To

Students are especially trying to figure out ways to separate themselves from the pack. Everybody goes to London and gets drunk . . . but not everybody works on water systems in Tanzania.

—Brandon Blache-Cohen, Amizade

"Karma Points": Motivations of Individual Volunteers

Many of us likely think "giving back" is the most common reason for international volunteering. A corporate employee volunteering in Haiti confirmed this view: "I understand that as a Caucasian American male born into the twentieth century, my lot in life is easier than 99.9 percent of all humans who have ever lived. I did not earn this; it was fate . . . the luck of the dice. If I can do something to help those who have a much harder lot, then I might have made the world a very slightly better place. And perhaps just slightly more fair."

There are, however, a wide variety of motivations, many far less altruistic than the conventional wisdom suggests. An American volunteer health professional in Ecuador who has gone on many service trips explained why he started: "I retired, and for the first year I was kind of aimless and didn't really know what was going on in my life and didn't have any purpose or direction. I did not want to commit to something long term. So this is very nice because it's a two- to four-week commitment; I like that aspect of freedom and not being tied down to something."

Motivations can be highly personal and far afield of even the most generous interpretation of what a desire to serve might look like. As an American working for a volunteer organization admitted, "Honestly, I went on the first brigade because I thought that the president of my university's chapter was very attractive."

As we saw earlier, student volunteers in particular are often focused on building their résumés.[1] Barrett Frankel, an American working in Rwanda, told me about volunteers who do so for reasons that mix that motivation with several others.

> I think many volunteers [especially college students] think that a trip to Rwanda makes for a great story and résumé content and come for less altruistic reasons. Some volunteers come to "fix" the world and think they can start with our Youth Village. They think their knowledge and/or skills are revolutionary and that in just a matter of days they can have a profound impact on changing the status quo. Other volunteers' reasons for coming are a bit more altruistic and they just want to lend a hand where needed, expose themselves to something a bit out of their comfort and knowledge zone, and learn something along the way.

This notion of giving back is worth some deeper exploration. Many volunteers, both domestic and international, use the phrase. It is something of an odd formulation; they are not giving back to those they believe directly provided the benefits they enjoy and for which, presumably, they are grateful. In a more fundamental sense, though, and supported by considerable historical evidence, giving back *does* fit, since many of the advantages people in wealthier communities enjoy resulted from past and current exploitation of poorer communities.[2]

It is unlikely, however, that an awareness of debt to formerly colonized countries whose raw materials and labor fed the prosperity of the industrialized nations is part of the reasoning. So, for volunteers, "paying forward" may be more apt; that notion seems to be at the core of the quote above from the self-described Caucasian American male.

Advertisements aimed at prospective volunteers are a valuable indicator of what the organizers believe to be the motivations that might lead people to volunteer. They use reports of returned volunteers and inspiring appeals: "She changed others' lives, and her own." "Students bring hope to Zambian village." "Make a difference." "The most awesome experience."

At its website, the Foundation for Medical Relief of Children (FIMRC)—which sends volunteers for short visits to seven countries—lists six reasons people should go on its trips, emphasizing the flexibility of schedule and type of program, lack of language requirement, and comparatively low cost. It also points to the professional advantages volunteering offers, something of great interest to many students: "Many of our volunteers go on to enroll in medical school, physician assistant and nursing programs, and other professional degrees. Often, they find that their volunteer experience is a point of interest during application interviews and provides them with a global background in the classroom. Medical professionals also appreciate our volunteer programs as an opportunity for professional development."[3] Clearly the emphasis is on advantages to be gained by the volunteers.

An organization in England that advocates for volunteering lists twenty-one reasons people volunteer.[4] This is not specific to international volunteering. Only four of the reasons seem to be about helping others directly, and none of those four show up at the top of the list. The top five are gaining new skills, knowledge, and experience; developing existing skills and knowledge; enhancing a CV; improving employment prospects; and gaining accreditation. Almost all twenty-one are about improving the volunteer's life, career, and social activities.

Missing from this list is another major reason for volunteering—the element of adventure, promoted by many organizations and tourist agencies that sponsor volunteer trips. Adventure even figures prominently in a 2006 article in the prestigious *Journal of the American Medical Association* about the opportunities for physicians in short-term international projects. The article's title is "Volunteering Overseas Gives Physicians a Measure of Adventure and Altruism."[5]

Adventure is at the center of the online announcement for a medical mission to Senegal in the accompanying box, which has much more information about the exotic and touristic nature of the trip than about the service element—and even that part is couched in terms of meeting "beautiful" and "enthusiastic" patients.

International Medical Relief Senegal Medical Mission, October 17, 2013–October 27, 2013

The pulsating culture of Senegal is easy to hear in their music and you will become immersed in their exciting culture with all of its richness from your first meal. You will hear them exclaim "kaay leck!" ("come eat!") as a bountiful plate with generous helpings of the local flavor is served for your whole group to share. The cultural traditions are rich with dance and song, yet one can certainly catch some shade under a majestic Baobab tree, also known as an ancient tree of life, which looks upside down.

This African country is the heart of where emotion meets adventure. You will be able to provide medical care in small, traditional African villages where enthusiastic patients will eagerly await their turn to greet you. The beautiful women with their multicolored dresses will come to clinic with exuberance typical of a bustling African market. Additionally the team will have the opportunity to provide greatly needed care to the Talibe youth. These young boys can be seen on the streets begging and most often go without any medical care.

INCLUDES SPECIAL TOUR TO WORLD HERITAGE SITE, GOREE ISLAND: You will also spend a day touring some of Senegal's most renowned sites, including the UNESCO World Heritage Site, Gorée Island. Here you can pay respects at the "doors of no return" on this historic slave-trading island. Whether you are enjoying the lively culture or music and dance or strolling on the famous white sand beaches, the colorful culture of Senegal will leave you with warm memories. Donation: $3450 www.international medicalrelief.org/medical-missions/senegal-2/.

The Internet is full of program descriptions like the one for Senegal that emphasize a country's beauty and exoticism, how the trip will contribute to the volunteer's life and career, and the satisfaction derived from service. Accompanying photos often show the (typically white) volunteers surrounded by smiling children and adult patients or community members (almost always brown and black). Given how pervasive these images are online in descriptions of volunteer trips, they must surely be part of what attracts prospective volunteers.

Of course, appeals to self-interest are not unusual in the world of volunteering. Scholars who study why people volunteer, domestically as well as internationally, have uncovered a wide variety of motivations that are similar to those listed by volunteering.org.[6] Psychologists have developed specific measures that identify broad categories of motivations; their studies focus on the variety of psychological goals that volunteers hope to achieve through volunteering.[7]

In fact, researchers studying volunteer activities have found altruism is only part of why people volunteer.[8] People are motivated as well by a desire for personal fulfillment and growth, sometimes by a desire for solidarity and justice, and even for social interaction and enjoyment.[9] One volunteer, reflecting this view, told me, "I think most of the people I know . . . do it to refresh their soul."

The Volunteer Functions Inventory (VFI), one of the most widely used measures of volunteer motivations, includes six sets of "functional motives": protective (from the difficulties of life); values (as ways to express altruistic and humanitarian values); career; social; understanding (to gain knowledge, skills, and abilities); and enhancement (of the ego).[10] Several studies of student volunteers that use the VFI rank "values" and "understanding" factors highest.[11]

Two other researchers constructed an inventory of twenty-eight altruistic, egoistic, social, and material-egoistic motivations to volunteer and found that volunteers "act not from a single motive or a category of motives but from a combination of motives that can be described overall as 'a rewarding experience.'"[12]

The mix of altruism and self-interest is not uncommon. Self-interest may shape the *choice* of activities through which people's desire to be helpful is expressed. "They tend," writes Robert A. Stebbins, "to gravitate only to those selfless opportunities within their targeted area of volunteering from which they believe they will reap valuable positive, personal, nonmaterial rewards such as experiencing pleasure, developing oneself (e.g., learning something, acquiring a new and valued skill), and expressing already-acquired skills and knowledge."[13]

Finally, among the individual motivations for volunteering, religion must again be mentioned. Religious faith or affiliation as a motive is not often studied explicitly, but the majority of volunteering, philanthropy, and international service by Americans is for religious institutions, so this demands attention. A study of 129 adult volunteers that used the VFI and added new open-ended questions found religiosity to be one of three additional motives not included in the original measure.[14] Church attendance and other forms of religious involvement can also be important predictors of the likelihood of volunteering.

A range of motives is also found in research on international volunteers, although these are often identified during or after the volunteer experience. For example, from open-ended interviews conducted with volunteers while they were participating in a medical-surgical clinic in Mexico, a researcher categorized motives as psychological benefits (essentially the personal satisfaction gained—what one person called "karma points"), career benefits, social interaction and camaraderie with other volunteers, opportunity to serve, and personal relevance.[15] In a study of alumni of two different international volunteer programs, participants mentioned five main motivations: have a challenging or meaningful experience; make a difference by helping others; gain greater cross-cultural understanding; travel or live abroad; and gain international experience and language skills.[16]

All in all, it is a complex mix of motivations that might lead a person to want to volunteer for an overseas health mission. Advertisers who appeal to potential volunteers' desire for self-development and adventure have a good basis in the scientific findings. They are aware they must appeal to the motives of the people they hope to recruit, and clearly this seems to work. The desire to give back is not the only motive, and it is often not the most important or even present at all.

"I Gained More Than I Gave": The Benefits for Volunteers

The primary benefit, for sure, is to the provider from the United States. There's not a person who does this, I think, who doesn't come away saying, "I feel better: one, because I'm able to do things I can't do in the United States; two, because maybe I've done some good; three, I've gotten to see another aspect of life." These are all conflated with each other. I think we all believe

we made the people we saw feel better for a period of time, but we're knowl-
edgeable enough to know that we haven't done a single thing to change the
context of their life. They're still poor; they're still living on the edge of sur-
vival sometimes. (American volunteer during one-week trip to Ecuador)

There is a widespread belief and some evidence that people who volunteer for
international programs do derive many benefits, similar to the expected gains
that motivate them.[17] They may gain experience and skills, knowledge of
other countries, career advantages, awards and praise, and great personal satisfaction.[18] Volunteering of all sorts, domestic and international, offers many
personal advantages and may even help alleviate depression and chronic
pain.[19] Sometimes it is a way to accrue college credits. No wonder so many
programs are promoted in terms of the personal benefits volunteers will gain
in confidence, skills, transformed outlook on life, and also a fun experience.

Many international volunteers say that they think they gained more
than they gave, and quite a few program organizers told me that even if
volunteers are not especially helpful to the communities where they work,
what they gain, and in some cases the financial support they provide for
ongoing programs, makes the effort worthwhile.

As we have seen, organizations often emphasize longer-term positive
effects for the volunteers when recruiting for overseas trips. The possibility that volunteer trips will be a "transformative experience" and inspire
future global health leaders is part of the rationale of some organizations
in planning trips.

One anticipated benefit is greater international and intercultural awareness and reduction in prejudice. Volunteers may develop a greater concern
about social justice and become more involved over their lifetimes in advocacy and social movements. A volunteer experience may be the impetus for
a choice later to pursue international service or some other international
career. Volunteers may make international connections and benefit from
social capital. And they can develop personal qualities or specific skills.
These are the claims at least. The benefits may be real, but the evidence for
them is still less than adequate.

Let's take a closer look at some specific benefits of volunteering.

Personal Satisfaction   Personal satisfaction is the subject of a great many
comments I recorded from volunteers, both in group sessions and in

individual conversations and interviews—even if it is rarely mentioned in the research. It is also a key factor motivating volunteers to repeat a mission: they enjoyed the previous experiences interacting with other volunteers and with patients.[20]

The representative of one organization, for example, recounts that volunteers often sign up for subsequent missions to Haiti. "They fall in love with the people. We have so many repeat people that come back, and back, and back, and back. It's unbelievable the return people."

In both missions I accompanied, the groups met twice to reflect together, and volunteers gave many examples of their excitement about the experiences. The group format for discussion—indeed, the group experience as a whole—appears to contribute to this enthusiasm. On our last night in Haiti, when the different teams all came back together for a barbecue, the group feeling was wonderful. We watched a video collage of photos from our time there set to great music, which reinforced the collective feeling of having had an awesome experience. There was lots of laughter and good feeling, along with expressions of dedication to doing good. One volunteer said, "When you leave Haiti, it's hard to talk about what you saw because people back home don't understand it, because it defied your expectations, it pushed you, it challenged you. It wasn't like what you thought it would be. But you have each other. There's eighteen people in this room, and you shared this together, so there will always be seventeen other people who understand what you went through."

Volunteers in Ecuador also spoke of their personal satisfaction at the final night's group meeting. "It's not often you spend eight days with forty people and you can honestly say unequivocally there's not one person that bugged you," said one. "You guys are all such kind souls and such wonderful people; hopefully I can stay in touch with you guys. You're really cool people. What went really well for me was I think every day I felt really fulfilled, every day was really worth the time and effort not just for myself but being able to see other people do the work that they do. Just being in this setting, Ecuador, is pretty amazing itself as well."

Said another,

> I guess for me the best thing is just a wonderful experience to get together with forty people and be able to connect like this and then get out there and really do something of value for these people in the villages. I'm used

to working in retail pharmacy day in and day out. I feel like I really don't do that much—mostly call insurance, with people bitching because they don't have their meds or their copays are a dollar. I'm thinking, "What am I doing?" It just gets to the point where I don't feel like I'm really making a difference in anybody's life, so this whole experience is really cool, because I feel like I got to do that.

Throughout the trips to Haiti and Ecuador, not only at last-night gatherings, I heard volunteers express their satisfaction with what they had experienced and with what they thought, perhaps with unwarranted optimism, they had accomplished. "Seeing a hundred patients a day for five days," said one, "you help improve the health potentially of a good number of people, like four hundred people or something like that. I like to contemplate this will have sort of ripple effects down the line. It's really rewarding to give a pregnant lady prenatal vitamins because the kid might have a better footing when they start out, that kind of thing. I just like the warm fuzzy feeling when you contemplate that kind of thing."

Another commented, "One good thing about the whole group is we're all kind of birds of a feather in that we want to kind of help people out. I just enjoy it; I really think we're helping people. I'm a little concerned that we're doing a little bit of damage in terms of ecological impact. So I have some complexes about flying 1,500 miles in a jet airplane and burning fuel and all that stuff. But the rest of it is just pure goodness helping people out. I really enjoy that part of it. I love the adventure part of it, seeing part of a foreign country, practicing a little Spanish."

A physician volunteer talked about the trip's effect on his feelings about his career. "When you do these sort of trips, it reminds you why you actually went into medicine. A lot of the time I think we get lost in our own worlds. I know I do very, very often. Sort of rush around and I think, 'Oh, God, I've got more patients to see.' And then I come out here and it takes about twenty-four hours to sort of come down to earth again and then today I realize that's why I went to school, that's why I'm still practicing medicine as I am. It's been really great."

And another spoke of a sense of renewal. "I come back feeling so energized and feeling so good because I not only get my little excitement rush from being out in this kind of environment, but you get the feeling, you know, that you've done something decent for humanity."

Representatives of sending organizations also hear this sense of personal satisfaction expressed by volunteers. "One of the main comments you get all the time when the volunteers come back," said one, "is 'Wow, I was actually living, you know, that purpose.' So that's fulfilling and rewarding."

"Everyone who goes comes back raving about it," a volunteer director for another sponsor organization told me, "which is really cool, because there's that immersive factor that volunteers really love. There's definitely a tremendous level of satisfaction that you get from knowing that each day you're doing something to benefit somebody else. I love that part of it."

Satisfaction and enjoyment are sometimes combined with gratitude for the privilege in their own lives, of which volunteers become very aware. Many talked about how being in a poor country increased their appreciation of their own good fortune. As one volunteer told me, "It kind of teaches me that I don't need to get upset about things that are so minor when you look at what some of the other folks in this world have and how much we have."

One volunteer reflected on a sense of solidarity with others that he gained from the experience. "It's not about me and them or me and us, but it's about we, and the symbiosis of all of us in this thing called life and the human experience. The best part is the kindness and compassion that define the people we've seen and all of you in the various different roles and paths in life. The essential experience of the interaction is really love and kindness, and it's very palpable, and that's why I keep coming back, because I like that feeling. I like learning from the people here, the indigenous people and from some amazing people in the brigade."

It's not surprising that short-term medical missions are so popular, with volunteers providing such glowing reports to their friends and colleagues when they return. Hearing (or reading online) about the joy of an international adventure with purpose and group solidarity makes these trips very attractive to prospective future volunteers.

International and Intercultural Awareness and Knowledge   Many believe volunteers gain greater international awareness and openness to other people as a result of their experiences, and that this helps reduce prejudice. Said one university official, "Awareness of other cultures, of cultural difference, of one's self, moving that transition from being ethnocentric to ethnorelative dramatically impacts the way people interact with other people."

While the limited research suggests these effects for some volunteers, it is based primarily on longer trips and tends to be assessed shortly after the volunteer's return. In one study of volunteers who had participated in social service or educational programs lasting either one, two, or eleven months (all of them longer than most short-term volunteer trips), more than 95 percent reported that international volunteering "increased their appreciation of other cultures, exposed them to communities different than the ones they grew up in, helped them gain a better understanding of the community where they worked, exposed them to new ideas and ways of seeing the world, and challenged their previous beliefs and assumptions about the world."[21] They also reported spending more time interacting with people from other racial and ethnic groups as a result of their experience.

Ben Lough and colleagues at the Center for Social Development at Washington University carried out one of the few studies that followed up with volunteers two to three years *after* their return. They found that both short- and longer-term volunteers self-reported more "international concern" than did a comparison group of nonvolunteers. There was no significant impact on self-rating of "intercultural relations." They concluded that volunteering may increase international awareness but perhaps no more than any other kind of international experience.[22]

Some organizations purposely try to break through volunteers' preconceptions. For example, Dr. Marjorie Muecke, assistant dean for Global Health Affairs at the University of Pennsylvania School of Nursing, emphasized the need for her students to recognize and learn from how people in other countries solve problems. "When our students go abroad, I want to change the notion of 'I'm going to save those poor and underserved people,' to 'You know what, I went to X country and guess what they're doing? It's so much better than what we are doing!' That is my goal in selecting places to visit while abroad. You can find examples in any country. You can find where people are doing things better than we are."

At its best, international volunteering can break down young volunteers' prejudices and dispel "simplistic and uninformed viewpoints about the countries and how people lived."[23] Volunteers tell of how "host communities were much more 'subtly different' than the crude representations of cultural difference they had gleaned from the media in their home country." In addition, some research suggests an increase in "global perspective" or even "global citizenship" among the volunteers, the majority of whom had never traveled outside wealthy countries and had a very limited understanding of the countries in which they had volunteered.[24] The evidence for these long-term effects from brief volunteer trips is slight at best and remains to be documented.

Later Involvement of Volunteers   Some organizations identify training future social justice advocates as one of their goals for volunteers. It is possible that international volunteering does increase overall participation in and commitment to advocacy, social movements, and social justice after the volunteer experience has been completed. In one study, 90 percent of former volunteers agreed their experience had increased their participation in cultural, environmental, or leisure activities, and many reported that their experience had particularly strengthened their commitment to both local and international volunteer service.[25] The study, however, followed the volunteers for only one month after their return. It also found that the effects of volunteering were greater in those who had participated in longer programs. The long-term implications for the more common brief volunteering are still to be demonstrated.

Preparing students for future advocacy is one of the goals of the university-based chapters of Timmy Global Health. Matt MacGregor emphasized the importance of the chapters in situating the volunteer experience in a much broader set of experiences that include engagement in the students' local community and education. They are "kind of like a congregation; once you go on the trip internationally, you come back and you're still participating in activities that support the programming with which you were involved, and that has much more potential in my mind to really have that kind of transformational impact on someone's attitudes and belief systems."

American Jewish World Service considers the formation of advocates a central goal of its volunteer programming. Sam Wolthuis, director of international operations, explains.

> The objectives of our short-term programs are to return from having been exposed to our partners all over the world and to mobilize and organize their communities here around an issue or campaign that AJWS is working on.

We think that volunteers who have been exposed to projects in the developing world and understand the complexities of HIV and AIDS because they've spent seven weeks working with an Ugandan NGO, they're in a position to come back and really advocate on behalf of that NGO with their communities here. We want them to do something with that impact, more than just change their major in college or go into international human rights or development ten years down the road. We want to see an immediate impact when they return, and we really emphasize that a part of that is to do something with the power and privilege that they hold just by being American citizens.

The goal of creating advocates is more than a hypothetical for AJWS; it is integrated into volunteer selection and preparation. "When they apply for those programs, we say, listen, you will have an obligation, a commitment, to this organization when you return," says Wolthuis, "so that even before you go, we're going to train you in how to mobilize and organize. We're going to train you in how to become community activists, in how to become an advocate on behalf of XYZ issue. And we start managing their expectations, so they know it's not just a one-week trip or experience or seven-week trip or experience."

Do AJWS volunteers become advocates as hoped? The evidence is still scant but is being studied. Says Wolthuis, "You hear volunteers return saying, 'I want to do something with that. I want to do something aside from just building this latrine' or 'I'm disappointed because I got much more out of it than I gave,' and we're saying, 'Great, so now you get to come home and do a lot more with that aside from just that latrine or that relationship.' We are a huge pipeline for aid donors, and the folks that sign our online petitions are often alumni. Many staff in the Jewish service world come from our alumni base."

Future International Careers and Service   Several researchers have found, and organizations report, that volunteering internationally increased the commitment of participants to international development and changed the course of their lives, including improving their employment prospects.[26] Medical trainees who had taken part in a global health experience reported greater knowledge of tropical medicine, were more likely to have changed their career paths toward general internal medicine and public health rather than subspecialty medicine or work in private practice, and were more likely to care for patients on public assistance or immigrants.[27]

There are many anecdotal examples of career changes. Brandon Blache-Cohen of Amizade spoke of how volunteering affects academics. "We actually found lots of faculty members we work with, I'd say 70 percent of them or 75 percent of them end up shifting their focus and research or taking on new research directly with the communities that we're partnering with. In fact, some of the best stories we have as an organization are about students we worked with twelve or fourteen years ago whose lives are changed enough that they went back to the region that we exposed them to, mastered the language, became tenured faculty members, and are now running programs with us again."

Ben Gleeson, an emergency medical technician from Kansas, told about how the volunteer experience had changed his thinking about his career path. "Being a paramedic, if I was going to make any transition to another healthcare field, I originally thought that there was no way that I would do anything outside of the emergency room. Primary care access was going to be way too slow and boring, it's the same thing over and over again. And then I came down here [to Haiti] and it really made me realize that primary care access can be an incredibly rewarding field, especially in underserved populations, which is where people are saying physician assistants really are needed."

Margaret Perko's experience volunteering in Uganda for several years affected her plans. She was a medical student at the University of Minnesota. "I wouldn't have done a master's in public health if I hadn't gone to Africa before medical school," she said, "but I see the value of doing the MPH. I really want to be working with people in public health and making people's lives better, not just treating them when they're sick. Now my goal is to be practicing in the United States ten to eleven months out of the year and then working long-term in a country, hopefully Uganda, on training physicians, working with the physicians, not just providing aid for a month, not just staffing a hospital for a month."

"I just was at a talk by an amazing woman who works in Somalia and Sudan," Matt MacGregor recounted, "and she was saying, 'I was going to be an Italian major and then I went on two Timmy trips and got really excited about both the good things they were doing and the bad things they were doing and the challenges they faced, and out of that I changed my career. I got really interested in international nutrition and now I've spent seven years at the World Food Program.' We know that a lot of our students are doing that."

Dr. Peter Fajans, formerly of the World Health Organization, reports that a great many staff members at WHO began as volunteers, "whether as part of an educational program or through some other mechanism." He also mentions summer internships at WHO, which "have probably been a launching pad for many careers in global public health." It is important to emphasize that some of these powerful experiences lasted for months, not the week or two that is more typical of volunteer programs today.

International Connections and Social Capital Networking and accruing social capital are important benefits for volunteers. They often report they have provided financial and other resources directly to people they met while volunteering and have used those contacts for future service trips or research projects.[28] Contacts made while volunteering may also be used to facilitate future employment opportunities or leverage resources for host communities.[29]

One example can be seen in a study of volunteers who participated in a ten- to fourteen- day Earthwatch Institute environmental research expedition that was conducted two months after their return. Developing new network ties while volunteering influenced their intent to participate in social movements, although it was too soon to have evidence for actual increases in participation.[30]

Specific Evidence of Benefits to Volunteers

Many of the assertions about the value of volunteer trips for the volunteers are based on anecdotes and a few short-term studies; it may be more ac- curate to speak of these benefits as *potential*. This does not mean the asser- tions are wrong, but it does mean that we still know very little about the longer-term impact of these trips and must be very cautious about making any claims regarding their value in changing lives.

A review of studies of medical electives for medical students in the United Kingdom, 40 percent of which were international, concluded that there was little solid evidence for claims that the experiences provided a wide range of potential benefits to the students in the areas of clinical knowledge and skills, attitudes, global perspective, personal and professional development, and institutional benefits. The review authors also found little systematic effort to create such an impact. They call these electives "missed opportunities."[31]

Margaret Sherraden and her colleagues at the Center for Social Development at Washington University have been in the forefront of developing evidence on the impact of service trips on volunteers. They summarize the effects as falling into several categories that overlap with those mentioned in the U.K. review: work experience and skills, personal development, intercultural competence and language skills, international knowledge and understanding, and civic and global engagement.[32] Notably, they repeatedly use the word "may" (which I've emphasized in these quotations) in describing what international volunteering accomplishes. For example, they write that it *"may* develop 'higher order' skills and abilities" and that "developing critical thinking skills *may* be accelerated." Volunteering *"may* contribute to employability" and *"may* contribute to personal and human development through heightened maturity, self-confidence, self-efficacy, self-awareness, and independence. Further, they write that "exposure to and interaction with people who are different *may* increase mutual understanding" and that international volunteering *"may* also result in greater knowledge and understanding of social, economic, and political issues in global context." Volunteers *"may* engage in civic learning that instills civic values and skills, and encourages future civic engagement" and "also *may* benefit personally from international social networks."

Sherraden and colleagues also cite sources suggesting negative effects or a lack of impact, but conclude, "The potential is high, therefore, for [international volunteering] to be a transformative experience in the lives of volunteers."

It is reasonable for scholars to be cautious about evidence, but this also suggests that we really are not very sure about the effects. It is clear from their review that the potential for long-term positive changes in volunteers is present, but the evidence is still in early stages of development. Even more challenging is to demonstrate that the entry of more Americans or Germans or Australians into international health careers improves the lives of people in the global South.

Gauging the Effects of International Volunteering Systematically

The International Volunteering Impacts Survey (IVIS) assesses the volunteer's perceptions of his or her international awareness, intercultural relations (i.e., interest in having relationships with people of other cultures and ethnic backgrounds); international social capital (referring to personal and organizational ties to people living in other countries); and international career intentions. Researchers used the IVIS in a study of two groups: 325 volunteers in one short and one longer program and 366 people who inquired about the programs but ultimately did not volunteer. The survey was administered both before and one week to one month after an international trip for those who traveled and in the same time frame for those who did not.

The two groups had comparable scores on all four dimensions of IVIS before the trip, but one month after the trip the travelers reported significantly greater international awareness, international social capital, and internationally related career intentions than the comparison group. It is unknown whether this change persists over a longer period of time.

The IVIS was also used with a random sample of 291 volunteers who mostly participated in education programs. They had gone to other countries either two or six years prior to the research by two different organizations, one whose program averaged four weeks and the other that sent volunteers for either two or eleven months. The results showed high levels of satisfaction as well as some impact on increased participation in cultural activities and volunteering and also on career goals, such that many volunteers reported being more committed to international development. The experience was also perceived as having improved their current and future employment, with those whose experiences lasted longer reporting a greater effect on their careers. (Lough, McBride, and Sherraden 2009a; McBride, Lough, and Sherraden 2012.)

Some researchers have begun to follow up over a longer period to determine whether immediate effects persist. An "alternative spring break" involving service in other countries was found to have a "huge impact" soon after the trip and continuing influence for some students a year later. But for some of the most enthusiastic students, the "experience had faded into a nice memory" after one year.[33]

In another example, students participated in a six-credit service-learning immersion program over winter break in Nicaragua, with an explicit social justice orientation that involved "raising consciousness about the historical development of racism, sexism, economic disparities, and unequal relations of power." The researcher included students who had participated over the course of five years and conducted interviews both with those who had just completed the program and with others further removed from their trips. He found important effects over time. Soon after returning, the students had new perspectives on the world: they were highly motivated to change their lifestyles and make a bigger difference. Most interesting, however, are the results of the longer-term follow-up: students had discovered that their initial plans for change were very difficult to achieve, given a variety of "personal, interpersonal, and institutional barriers associated with their lives in the United States." Some did become activists and/or change their career plans, but for many it was difficult to talk about their new consciousness with skeptical friends and family members, and they experienced considerable conflict about making changes in their lives.[34]

The studies suggest that the benefits anticipated for international volunteers are hardly guaranteed and may be difficult to achieve. Longer stays do seem more likely to produce such results, and there is some evidence that living with a host family and use of "guided reflection" can contribute to greater intercultural competence.[35]

Potential Negative Effects on Volunteers

There are also potential negatives for the volunteers. For instance, they may face travel-related safety risks. They may become ill, most commonly in the form of gastroenteritis (the infamous "traveler's diarrhea" or "Montezuma's revenge"). Roads and vehicles in poor condition and poorly regulated driving increase the chances of traffic accidents. And volunteers have on occasion been the victims of crime—including rape.[36]

But a more general concern for volunteers across the board is that they may return home with perceptions of the host country and of development in general that are misguided and simply wrong. Kate Simpson's analysis of marketing materials directed toward British students who can afford to volunteer internationally during a "gap year" between high school and university applies as well to much shorter-term programs.

> The gap year produces . . . a construction of the world where there are simplistic boundaries between two places i.e. that of the north and south, that perpetuates a simplistic ideal of development. This ideal in turn legitimizes the validity of young unskilled international labour as a development "solution." . . . Gap year projects create a publicly accepted "mythology" of development. . . . Indeed, the very legitimacy of such programmes is rooted in a concept of a "third world," where there is "need," and where European young people have the ability, and right, to meet this need.[37]

She adds,

> The dominant ideology is that doing something is better than doing nothing, and therefore, that doing anything, is reasonable. . . . Throughout gap year literature and publicity there are multiple references to the "usefulness" of volunteers, and how they will be "needed" by the communities or environments in which they work. [One] quotation . . . promises "a culture older than Genghis Kahn needs you!" This statement, made seemingly without irony, implies that Mongolia is crumbling for want of a few British teenagers.[38]

Lauren Wallace agrees, asserting that volunteering by premedical students, not unlike other voluntourism projects, is governed by a rhetoric of "good intentions," "need," and "making a difference." Health improvements, in this view, mostly require the work of groups of semitrained but enthusiastic visitors.[39]

Simpson also warns that volunteer exposures can serve to reinforce stereotypes or create new ones. This includes the common "poor but happy" conclusions that so many people come to, based on so little evidence. As a volunteer in Haiti told me, "We have everything and are unhappy, and they have nothing but are happy." This view falsely generalizes about an entire nation and may conveniently, if unintentionally, serve the function of excusing or accepting poverty because it doesn't really bother poor people.

I also heard other volunteers voice astonishingly simplistic generalizations about the people in their host countries. In a group meeting after two days of clinics, volunteers spoke of Ecuadoreans as all being grateful, kind, gentle people who are less stressed than Americans. It struck me as quite incredible that people could make such broad assumptions based on two days of brief encounters in a clinic environment with mostly sick people whose lives the volunteers knew nothing about and whose language they did not understand.

One said, for example, "I don't think these people have the same fear of being insecure that Westerners or especially Americans have. Americans are very afraid they're going to lose this; they're afraid they're going to lose that. And these people live life day to day. They see things that we can hardly imagine seeing, and it's just part of life."

Said another, "I think all of us have been impressed by the fact that the people we've seen in the last few days are almost to a person, I would call them sweet, gentle souls. They're a delight to talk to. They're a delight to listen to, and a delight to lay hands on. I think that's one of the privileges that many of us enjoy [as physicians]."

And a third, "They're such kind and gentle souls. They're not wrapped up in bullshit that most of us are, and I am, in the States. It just humbles you and it's just wonderful, because these people, you look in their eyes and you know, they appreciate the hell out of what we're doing."

Another volunteer was pretty sure what the patients he saw would remember of this brief encounter: "I think they'll never forget us. They'll appreciate it always. It feels great."

One more example of this "benign" stereotyping: "I came here to learn from them about what truly being human is, in their very unique, humble, innocent, grateful way."

Two of the interpreters—both Americans who had lived in Ecuador for more than a year—spoke with me about how upset they were by these generalizations. They had lived in the country long enough to realize

Ecuadoreans are as diverse as any other people and that such sweeping statements are uninformed and misleading. This contrast between the new arrivals and Americans with more experience in the country underlines the problem of many short-term volunteers thinking they have learned something important when it is impossible to have more than superficial impressions, often incorrect ones, after a few days.

Sadly, these comments support Simpson's contention about the development of stereotypes and the conclusion that a few foreigners are what is needed to change people's lives.

In Appendix B, I offer some guidelines for prospective volunteers, including the recommendation to associate with a reputable organization that has procedures in place to maximize the preparation and well-being of volunteers.

There is no doubt that many volunteers feel strongly that their experience on an international health mission changed their lives. For some, it truly does. One brief experience may lead to another, longer overseas trip and even blossom into a career in international or local service. It is certainly the case that most volunteers report great satisfaction with the work they have done and the people they have met. But the fact remains that there is little evidence that short-term volunteer trips produce the kinds of transformational changes that are often promised.

Most studies are carried out soon after volunteers return, so a claim of lifelong changes is yet to be well documented. The study of volunteers who went to Nicaragua in particular suggests caution about such claims, since the researcher found that initial enthusiasm and intention to change usually diminished markedly over time.[40] Much more long-term follow-up research is needed for organizers to be able to claim, as some do, that even if volunteers don't make much difference in host communities, at least they will be influenced to make important contributions to justice over the long term.

Many people involved in international volunteering believe strongly that its value is in great part the contribution it makes to influencing people to be more educated global citizens with a commitment to social justice in the future. This is a noble goal; whether it can be achieved through short-term volunteering programs remains to be shown. It would be valuable to know not only what changes occur, specifically, but also which types of experiences are most likely to have positive effects. The best evidence so far seems to suggest that preparing for the experience through critical readings and discussion before the trip and following up with reflections afterward, as well as increasing the length of stay, may help maximize the impact.

Those who defend brief volunteer trips as transformative in positive ways for the volunteers and as therefore creating future advocates for the poor, even if they do not contribute anything to the host community in the short run, bear a responsibility to show that this is truly the case. They also should be considering how to address volunteers' beliefs that they have truly made a difference when the evidence for this, as we shall see, is also very limited. Hoping it is so does not make it happen.

Part III

The Host Communities

If the massive investment in short-term health programs is to be justified, it must be in terms of the value to the third and most important party in this picture—the host communities. In the next few chapters I look more carefully at the advantages and disadvantages that short-term volunteer programs bring to the communities they are intended to benefit. In doing so, I rely on existing studies but also on what people who work in host countries say about the volunteers and programs they encounter in their daily activities. They tell us a great deal about what types of volunteers are most appreciated (and which are not) and what types of programs are most valuable. They help us weigh the arguments on each side of the debate about short-term volunteering.

5

The Best and the Worst

Host Perspectives on Volunteer Programs

I really appreciate the volunteers and we are proud of them. We welcome
them with open arms.
— Hospital staff member in Niger

I've never seen the contribution; they only waste our time. Some of them feel
like when they come down here, they think they know it all, they have seen it
all, and that is no good.
— Hospital staff member in Ghana

More important than the value of medical missions or brigades to the
organizations and volunteers is the impact on host communities. Although
many people from sending countries have written extensively about the
benefits and problems of volunteer programs, there has been very little attention given to the views of people in the host-countries who receive volunteers. The two quotes above reveal how widely disparate host views may
be: some welcome volunteers, while others think they have little, no, or
even negative value.

Interviews with fifty-five host-country staff members in four countries
are revealing. They talked about their experiences working with volunteers, the advantages and disadvantages of volunteer programs, and how
those programs might best meet the needs of their countries. In an earlier
chapter you read some of what they think volunteers should know before
arriving in their countries. Here you'll read more about what they think

makes a good or bad individual volunteer and what they consider evidence for the value of volunteer programs.

In addition to the perspectives of staffs from the host countries, I also include insights from "expatriates"—people who have worked or are currently working full-time in host countries and have had two or more years of experience with volunteers in those countries. This was a good opportunity to gain their perspective as well on the benefits and drawbacks of having short-term volunteers work in their programs. These expatriates include physicians, country staff for U.S. NGOs, and community development workers; most are Americans, with a few from France and Latin America.

Host-country perspectives truly do run the gamut when it comes to assessing the value of volunteers. For instance, asked what volunteers contribute, an Ecuadorean doctor said, "Their energy, technical capacities, and their eagerness to volunteer. They are not egotistical. Volunteerism, for me, is being closer to God. We have not seen any difficulties. Actually, only benefits. Our nurses learn from those nurses that come, and our doctors learn from those doctors. And the volunteers learn our characteristics."

Of course, the same hosts who speak so positively often have very particular criticisms, as you'll read later. And they are very clear about what distinguishes between the best and the worst volunteers.

"Good" and "Bad" Volunteers

"The volunteers I like are very open to the culture and very curious about what's going on in the country," a Ghanaian host staff member responded to a question about the qualities of "good" and "bad" volunteers. "They try to adapt themselves to the place. I'm totally, totally sure that the majority of the volunteers that I have seen are that type—very open, curious, and very interested in how can you learn from that place. The ones that I don't like mainly believe in the superiority of one culture over another one. [They are the ones who think,] 'We are more civilized people than you and because of that it would be a good idea to help you to become more civilized.'"

A Haitian clinic staff member made a very interesting characterization. "A bad volunteer isn't a volunteer," he said. "In effect, it's someone who just visits and wants to be a tourist. A real volunteer is someone who wants to help and who does all he can to help. I remember having an experience with one volunteer. I had the responsibility just to take them from the clinic to the volunteer center, not to go anywhere else. But on the way there, he wanted to go to a place just to drink something. I didn't want that, so he was very angry, but I had no choice just to do what I had to do."

Said a staff member from Ecuador, "Those are the type of volunteers that I don't really like. There are some that are really high-maintenance, as you say in the United States; they don't really want to lose their comfort when they come here. And of course, for the places that we visit, it's kind of rough sometimes."

From the interviews, it is possible to articulate specific characteristics that make for a good or bad volunteer. For instance, good volunteers are *willing to work hard and do whatever needs to be done.* "The volunteers really help us here in Haiti—really, really," said a Haitian nurse. "They really bring us Haitians a lot of help. When they come, they work a lot. They work a lot, a lot."

A hospital staff member in Niger described one particular volunteer who seems to have embodied this idea of doing whatever needs to be done. "From the moment she arrived at the hospital, she was curious about everything. She was interested in everything. When she saw the patient's relative doing laundry, she helped wash [clothes]. When the children were playing, she played with them. When we were unloading a truck, she helped."

The best volunteers, said a Ghanaian nurse manager, "are punctual, hard-working, respectful, and they have the knowledge, too." And a Haitian laboratory technician remarked, "I see a volunteer as someone who really comes to help, so he wasn't forced, who comes and is at ease, who works well with others and with a lot of determination. He is very participative and determined."

A second characteristic of a good volunteer is that she or he has *good interpersonal skills.* A woman who works in administrative support at the CURE hospital in Niger gave "a lot of importance" to two criteria: "openness and good listening skills." Another in Niger said, "They get along well with the patients."

Several staff members specifically mentioned that a good volunteer is *adaptable.* From a medical resident in Ghana: "Adaptability. Ability to adjust to the culture, to the people." And from an American doctor in Niger: "The best quality is flexibility. Things almost never go as planned on a trip like this. It helps to roll with the punches."

A different American doctor, this one in Nepal, also mentioned adaptability. "The main issue," he said, "[is a volunteer's] willingness and ability to adjust to local living standards such as no water, no heat and no electricity, and to cultural norms. For example, a single female disappearing on the back of a motorbike with a single male to an adjacent town would be majorly frowned upon."

Many of the staff members characterized good volunteers as those who come with *technical skills*. "I saw a surgeon I liked a lot because of his competence," a nurse in Niger told Susan Rosenfeld. "He was very quick and efficient. He operated on several children a day, sometimes five, and he did it alone. I hope his team comes back."

The issue of skills relates directly to the motivation of volunteers. A medical resident in Ghana characterizes good volunteers this way: "They are actually skilled in what they do and are not just here to gain some experience they wouldn't have gained where they were." An Ecuadorian social worker agrees that volunteers who arrive with experience and skills are the best: "We do not have sufficient human resources and they are a big help with the work. For example, the volunteer that speaks Spanish and has experience of the work and life—the aid and effect she has on the community is much larger than the one a student would make. The youth have their curiosity and eagerness, but the experienced already bring what they can teach and what they can use to help."

The final characteristics of good volunteers, according to hosts, are that they are *humble and respectful*. "I think that among all professionals there needs to exist what we call habitual humility," said a Haitian physician. "It's a good thing to develop."

A Ghanaian medical resident concurred, mentioning "the ability to learn, to be humble, nonjudgmental, but to make honest criticism where that demands it." He continued, "Basically, I think the best volunteers would be the ones who respect the whole system, respect the people they are working with and then also have a good understanding."

"Empathy requires hard work," writes Dr. Jack Coulehan. Coulehan is emeritus professor of preventive medicine and senior fellow of the Center for Medical Humanities, Compassionate Care, and Bioethics at Stony Brook University. "Without the wisdom of humility, altruistic behavior can lead to self-delusion, compassion can become an obsession, and both may generate a damaging sense of hubris."[1] While these words were written for physicians working in the United States, they are no less applicable to health-related volunteer work in poor countries.

I witnessed a startling example of hubris from a nonphysician on one of the volunteer trips. A new type of record system involved writing numbers on patients' arms and entering their personal information into a laptop. I asked the system's creator whether patients in the host community would be OK with these new and unfamiliar procedures. He laughed my question off, almost scoffing. "Not a problem," he said. "They'll do it. It's the gringo aura; they'll do whatever we tell them."

That kind of attitude, from someone who had spent quite a lot of time in the country and worked very hard to develop the record system, can only diminish the value of all the hard work. The idea that people will go along because we gringos tell them to has been at the heart of many failed programs around the world.

To sum up the good characteristics, here's what the medical director of a hospital in Niger said. "The ones with the highest ratings would be those who keep coming back and those who have a skill that is needed at the hospital. For example, there is a married couple who are retired doctors. One is a surgeon and the other an ob-gyn. They can now hit the ground running and know how to live in the area and manage their daily life."

Descriptions of "bad volunteers" centered on three main characteristics that are, not surprisingly, the flipside of qualities ascribed to "good volunteers." The first is that bad volunteers demonstrate an *unwillingness to follow rules or carry out assigned duties*. A Haitian employee of Heart to Heart International told me that some volunteers even occasionally refuse their assignments.

An American expatriate in Haiti described the problem posed by volunteers who don't follow the program's rules. "Rules are pretty clear when it comes to the clinics. You cannot go into the pharmacy. You are a volunteer. The pharmacy belongs to the Haitian pharmacist. There is a system. You may not agree with it 100 percent, but it works better. We've been doing this for two years and about six months now, and this is the best thing we've come up with for not having a computer, for not having a shared inventory system. Don't touch it! And it's a really hard thing. Once, twice, three times a month I'm dealing with somebody who's got an itchy hand and wants to go in the pharmacy and rearrange things."

Then there are bad volunteers, often know-it-alls, who are *bossy and not respectful*. As a Ghanaian nurse administrator said, "They don't take our advice, or if you tell them something, they think they know better than us and that is not good."

Some volunteers act in an "autocratic" way, said another Ghanaian who works with women in labor. "What they say is final. You just have to take it. That's what I don't like about them." A Haitian physician concurred. "If you're trying to arrange it your way, like you're an American and you come, 'Oh, in the States, here's the way we do it; it's best to do it that way,' and you obviously want to help, but you're going to mess it up. The ones who want to impose their own way, and if someone would like to do so, well it would be a problem for our field staff, and they will report to us about that, and they would not like that at all. And it would not be fit to come and try to impose your own way." A staff member in Niger made a similar comment about the need for humility and respect: "Observe first before commenting. Not 'why are you doing that?' Wait a little while."

You can add arrogance to being autocratic. A Ghanaian hospital employee was especially frank: "The most difficult task is they don't understand our system, especially the white ladies who come here. When they come here there are systems here, so you must understand each department and what he does and when he does and how he does it. So they come here, they didn't normally understand us. They just think they have done something at the top [of the Ghanaian hospital hierarchy], so they don't care about those who are down."

The short-term nature of the visits is a factor, too. "Try not to replace the local doctor, because you're going to leave," says a Haitian staff member. "Try not to replace the one in the pharmacy. Try not to organize the pharmacy your way because you are going to leave."

Barret Frankel, an American expatriate who has received and worked with many short-term volunteers in a youth village in Rwanda, summed up the views expressed by many hosts. "Many volunteers come expecting to teach something new or improved and do not respect the fact that many ways of thinking and operating have served the people just fine for decades and even centuries. Are there more efficient ways of cutting the lawn than using machetes? Of course, but machetes get the job done just the same."

The third characteristic frequently mentioned to describe a bad volunteer is a *lack of communication skills or cultural understanding*. "They should know more Spanish," said an Ecuadorean community health worker. "It makes it a little more difficult for us to communicate with them. And they hardly understand us."

Not all comments about communication, though, are specific to knowledge of the local language. Many hosts remarked about the words volunteers choose to use.

"Not Twi [a language of Ghana], but the language, how they relate with us," says a Ghanaian. "Normally, let me put the 'white woman' and 'white man' in quotes, when they come, they look down upon the black people, they think we are fools and monkeys so they do anything anyhow. So I would say the language, how they communicate, how they relate with us. They don't understand us."

As for cultural norms, comments from hosts fall along a wide spectrum. For example, a hospital social worker in Niger says, "There are some who try to dress like us, but there are others who stay as they would at home. For example, shorts. Women in shorts!"

In addition to the characteristics described by host staff members, there are others that fall in the category of inappropriate or even illegal behavior. Some volunteers use the trip as an opportunity to drink and/or use drugs and then can't do the work the next day, and there are those who arrive seeking sexual liaisons with people in the host communities. These were mentioned only by American expatriates and volunteers and not by host-country staffs. But it is worth noting that such things do occur and can cause difficulties for everyone involved.

One American who works full-time with hundreds of volunteers in a host country compared the good ones who arrive after reading about the country and are willing to follow directions with the much more rare ones he wants to send home. The latter may be there because they felt pressured by others or thought it would be romantic. "Volunteering isn't romantic," he notes. "It's dirty. And if you can't stand to be dirty and dusty and uncomfortable, then you should just go to Montego Bay."

Evidence of Benefit

Anecdotal evidence of good and bad individual volunteers and programs is relatively easy to come by in interviews. Seeking more specific information, I asked host-country staff members *how* they know whether volunteers make a difference for patients and the communities where they work. And I asked them for evidence that might document their impact.

"We get to know if the volunteers are making an impact if we see the import of their visit after they're done," a Ghanaian hospital employee told me. "If they give us feedback on what they've done, if we get to either read a paper on what they've done or see physical structures they put in place—for example, the fetal assessment center that we have over here." An Ecuadorean district official cited some specifics he thought offer proof of value: "Evidence from the execution of the brigades, the agreements, the history of each of the communities and clinical follow-ups, and the hospital records. And especially from the living testimony of those who have improved in health."

A Haitian doctor told me he relies on reports from local residents to assess the value of volunteers: "From the report I have from people in the field, they are good people, because you know when they go in the field and work, people in the field, the local people, will be reporting to us how the person is."

Finally, a staff member in Niger also did not rely on evaluations; rather, "for the cleft palates, the proof is the photos."

Every host-country staff member was asked to rate, on a scale from 0 to 10, the overall value of having volunteers come to their countries. The combined rating by the fifty-two who answered was 8.16: by country, it was Ecuador, 8.9; Niger, 8.85; Haiti, 7.63; and Ghana, 6.75. Some indicated they might have given an even higher score, but because nothing is perfect, they did not feel comfortable saying 10.

Even when they mention undesirable qualities, most host-country staff members value volunteers a great deal and say there are few bad ones. It's important to note that many owe their jobs, at least in part, to the presence of volunteers, and that an American interviewer may be perceived as working for the volunteer organization—even though neither I nor any of my research associates were. The responses may reflect some understandable caution. The value of the observations comes from the staff members' familiarity with volunteers and their willingness to cite concerns even to someone from the outside and despite their allegiance to the organization that sponsors or hosts volunteers.

The four groups of host-country workers differed in terms of their financial relationships to the outside organization and also in terms of the interview situation. Thus it is not surprising that the Ghanaian staff members gave volunteers the lowest score and made some of the most obviously negative comments (for example, about the attitudes of white people toward Africans). They are hospital employees who do not depend on volunteer sponsors for their living, and they are more likely to work with volunteers who come for research rather than to provide services. Most important, perhaps, they were interviewed by a Ghanaian American fluent in their local language and therefore probably felt they could be more open.

Even so, some Haitian staff members were also critical overall in their comments, despite being interviewed by a white American and having jobs largely funded by the American volunteer organization. The fact that many of them are highly trained and have had a great deal of experience with unskilled volunteers who have flocked to their country, especially since the earthquake, is certainly relevant.

Volunteer Length of Stay

One issue that comes up repeatedly with host-country staff members is the length of time volunteers spend in their countries. They report that the volunteers have stayed for a week or two on average, much as sending organizations indicated. A few stay longer.

There was a remarkable amount of consensus about what would work best. "Three weeks seems ideal to me," an Ecuadorean physician told me, and a staff member in Niger agreed, saying, "I think at least three weeks. I imagine it is during the vacation so three weeks to a month. That depends. The surgical teams come for one week but they work hard. It depends on what area."

A social worker at the Niger hospital said, "I think that a volunteer can come for a minimum of a month. For less than a month it is difficult to explain what a volunteer should do." Another man in Niger agreed, "Two weeks we can do something. Three weeks we can do something. One month we can do something. But two or three days, no." For the most part, visits of only one or two weeks are considered inadequate.

A Haitian nun assisting at a rural clinic goes even further. "If you have a doctor for a week or two weeks, they do not have time to do everything." When I asked her what would be ideal, the answer was a year.

The medical director of a hospital in Niger agreed that "the longer, the better." He said, "A year would be fantastic. Two months is very good; they are more helpful the second month." Why are they more helpful the second month? As another man from Niger, who works in the hospital laboratory, observed, "The first month they are culturally lost; you need a month to adapt."

These comments reflect agreement across the four countries that to accomplish anything, most volunteers have to spend more time getting to know the work and the environment; ideally, they would stay for at least three or four weeks. A Haitian nurse concurred, saying one month would be best. However, another Haitian, an interpreter working with volunteers, acknowledged that that might not be realistic. "Sometimes when the volunteer doctors come in, they say they don't really have vacation, they just ask for one week off, two weeks' vacation. That's all they can do. They cannot stay for long. Even though we like to have them work for more than one week, they can't. We cannot do anything about that."

It is interesting to note, however, that, as a Haitian physician who has worked with many volunteers and organizations observed, a volunteer who stays *too* long might become arrogant and uncooperative as a result. "I would not allow more than one month," he said. "When a person starts working, that person may be humble, may follow all the rules, but after one month, two months, that person may think, oh I know everything about [the organization] now so I can do this, I can do that and I can just break the rules. Or they might say, 'OK, after one month, because I am a volunteer, they can't fire me, so I can do whatever I want.' It's always better to have new people come." This was an unusual comment but reflects the important concerns discussed earlier about volunteers who assume they know best and do not cooperate with the host staff.

Host-country staff members want volunteers to stay long enough to be more effective than they can be in a week or two, but at least one expressed the view that they should not stay so long that they take over. There are some differences by country. In Niger, they all want volunteers to stay longer if possible; these host staffpersons work at a faith-based children's hospital that receives a small number of volunteers, many of them for surgical "camps." In Haiti, by contrast, there is wariness about the role of the volunteer in relation to Haitian staff members. Unlike Niger, Haiti has received many thousands of volunteers in recent years and also has many more of its own physicians.

There are only a few other studies that have actually asked host-country staffs what they think about short-term volunteers. Two of them, focused on physicians, found much more negative attitudes. Dutch researchers discussed international volunteering with eight experienced physicians from sub-Saharan Africa who were studying international health in Antwerp. These professionals considered volunteers mostly inexperienced, unskilled, and unprepared, both culturally and professionally, and often not willing to value local staff expertise. They did, however, report positive experiences with volunteers who stayed longer and tried to learn the language, brought supplies, trained others in specific skills, and were willing to work in remote areas. These "good" volunteers were appreciated for improving access to care and providing a "concrete expression of international solidarity."[2]

Similar results emerged from Namibia. In interviews with nine health-care professionals affiliated with the Namibia School of Medicine, researchers found concerns about volunteers' lack of cultural understanding of the country, which resulted in their offending people and making visits ineffective. Attitudes of superiority and wanting to impose or teach their own methods and opinions in ways that were inappropriate to the environment were also troubling. They write, "Participants also perceived visiting health care professionals as attempting to impose their visions of health and health care onto the local environment. Local health care professionals felt that visitors were often trying to apply Western concepts of medicine and standards of care in a setting where resource limitations often make such concepts impossible to implement. The local health care professionals acknowledged that although the ideas brought by visitors were good, they were rarely relevant in the environmental context."[3] Nevertheless, these Namibians welcomed international volunteers who were willing to make a commitment to their country in a spirit of partnership and mutual respect.

My interviews included a wider variety of people working with volunteers, and they were quite positive overall about the advantages of having volunteers from other countries. Even when they referred to problems, most of them expressed appreciation for those who arrived willing to work hard, to learn, and to respect local practices; these attitudes were similar to the opinions physicians expressed in other studies. They especially valued the volunteers who brought needed skills and who expressed caring for patients.[4]

"What distinguishes the very best [volunteers]," said a staff member in Niger who acts as a liaison between the hospital and NGOs that send volunteers, "is the openness of spirit. Opening their heart to the staff, to other people. Talking about things, remarking about things, without judging."

Host-country staff members also believe volunteers should be well informed about the country and the work before they arrive and should stay for about a month so they have sufficient time to adapt to the work environment. Most organizations, however, cannot or do not send volunteers for that long, and most do not provide much in the way of cultural preparation.

We still do not know whether even the best volunteers and programs produce better health outcomes in measurable ways. In the next chapters, which explore some of the positive and negative effects on or costs to host communities of having volunteers, we begin to get closer to an answer.

6

Benefits to Host Communities

"They saw a lot of people," a Haitian man who provides logistical support for Heart to Heart International volunteers told me, speaking of a recent brigade of volunteers. "I think that people are really satisfied when they have people like this coming, doctors, surgeons, specialists."

It stands to reason that a well-designed and executed volunteer trip should benefit the host communities, the sponsoring organizations, *and* the volunteers themselves. At issue is what we really know about the impact on communities of short-term health volunteering. There is precious little systematic research on this question, and organizations rarely attempt to collect evidence of their impact.

In surveys and interviews, we asked all the organizers, volunteers, and host-community staff whether volunteers make a difference and for any evidence they have of the value to host communities. Most mentioned examples of positive effects, but they were primarily anecdotal or based on observation, with a focus on "inputs," such as number of staff members employed and amount of money spent, or on "outputs" such as number of people who participated in a clinic or how much health-related educational material was distributed. But some also focused on actual "outcomes"— that is, measurable changes in the lives of host-community members. Taken together, they provide valuable examples of positive contributions made by volunteer-sponsor organizations.

We have seen that the organizations focus on health-related goals at the same time as other goals. The benefits to host communities, as reported by local staff, organizers, and volunteers alike, can also be divided into those that are and those that are not specific to improving health.

Health Benefits to Host Communities

Extra Hands and Energy   A common and entirely understandable response to the question about the benefit of volunteers is that they provide additional help to local organizations that are almost always understaffed. Hospitals and clinics with very few trained staff members are often overwhelmed by the variety of tasks that at facilities in wealthier countries are taken care of by nursing assistants, clerical support staff, and people in a wide variety of occupational categories. Additional health professionals can make it possible to see more patients, and unskilled volunteers can assist with paperwork and some aspects of intake.

There is often great appreciation for volunteers who alleviate the burden of these tasks. A Haitian man who helps run one of the Heart to Heart clinics told me that volunteers provide a benefit

> because we have more hands. So if we don't have any volunteers, we have only one doctor working, we have to reduce the number of the patients, but imagine we have volunteers and among them we have three medical doctors or two medical doctors, more people will be seen, more patients will come. So the advantage of the presence of the volunteers [is] we have more people to see the doctor, and the work is done faster.
>
> When they come they help us, and since our staff still isn't very big, they help us especially in the pharmacy and with triage work, like you see today. So they help us in every way.

"Proof that shows that the volunteers are working?" A security guard at the CURE hospital in Niger repeated Susan Rosenfeld's question and then responded, "I'll give you an example. Physical therapy. Without a volunteer in this area the physical therapist can see maybe four or five patients, but with a volunteer physical therapist maybe eight or nine patients. That's a big help that the volunteer brings." Said another hospital staff member, "The more there are volunteers, the more our tasks are lessened." As a full-time American physician in Niger explained, "The right kind of volunteer relieves stress and lightens the load of the long-termers."

Josh Jakobitz, operations officer in Haiti for Heart to Heart International, has a perspective that goes beyond extra hands to embrace the idea of energizing the existing staff. "A lot of what [the volunteers] do I think sometimes is just motivation. Like they come, they're fresh, they're enthused, they're working alongside the Haitians. Honestly, we've been doing this for over two years and we do the same thing week after week after week after week. We work in the same places, the un-air-conditioned clinic in Bellaire, the un-air-conditioned clinics in Léogâne, dirty roads, the same commutes, and so I think that a lot of their energy gets transferred to the teams. They pick up on it."

Medicine, Equipment, and Supplies   Many program sponsors ask volunteers to purchase supplies in advance or carry in their luggage medications and other equipment supplied by the organization. Thus volunteers are valued sometimes as much for what they bring with them as for their own presence. "Volunteers bring their knowledge, their participation," said a nurse in Niger. "They also bring [medical] products with them . . . brand new products the country doesn't have yet."

A Haitian man who helps run a Heart to Heart clinic said he especially values the free medicine. "The price is low compared to other labs, and medicines you might buy for a lot of money, they have been almost free. If I'm sick, I can have the doctor see me, so I think this is a good thing giving this expensive medicine free to people, which they would buy for a lot of money, so this is something good."

Needed equipment is highly valued. "Some of them, they can help, like the monitors and other gadgets that we need to care for the patients," said a woman who has administrative duties at the university hospital in Kumasi, Ghana. "Improvement of the work, there are improvements after the volunteers."

Training and Capacity Building   It is difficult to document, but volunteers often create or reinforce local institutions in ways that allow the institutions to provide better services. For instance, FAVACA focuses on sending consultants to work with organizations that request them for specific purposes. As Chris Beyer of FAVACA recalls,

> One project in particular that has changed both the health aspect as well as the civil laws of the country has been in Antigua, where we had a volunteer who works with individuals suffering domestic and particularly sexual assault. She has been working with both the government and the health institutions there to create a facility so that people who have been assaulted can go and get the proper medical documentation that they have been raped or assaulted. This individual has been able to work with the government to get some laws instituted as well as setting up a facility and teaching nurses how to go about collecting all the necessary evidence . . . and then also working with prosecutors to figure out how they can start moving many of these cases.

Training staffers to be able to accomplish their work and meet professional goals more effectively is an important facet of capacity building. One part of the Becton Dickinson Volunteer Service Trips has involved creating and equipping laboratories; in Haiti, the company also trained laboratory workers from both public and private laboratories in several regions of the country in procedures for good laboratory management.

My student Ana Arteaga and I spoke with an official of the Haitian Ministry of Health, who explained, "I attended these training sessions and thought everything was well done, and in my conversations with the participants they pointed out the quality of the training, that the level is very fitting for them. After a training session, we have lots of useful training, very important for the laboratory. I think that it's an activity worth developing because the sharing of ideas is very useful. When many people are thinking up ideas, each one will improve his own idea and come up with a better one."

We asked one of BD's volunteer laboratory trainers how she knew whether her work had made a difference. She told us she could see it in the responses from the students. "Last week, somebody was asking if we're coming back next year, because she would like to attend, and wanted to know how to guarantee that she's going to be in the class next year. She wants her name on the list, she wants to make sure that she's the one picked from her lab. And the gratitude expressed at the end of the week, they're grateful for what it is that we're able to share with them."

The trainer continued.

For example, today, for our class, we had the two people from Partners in Health who attended the BD training last March. They came back and showed this group an SOP [development of Standard Operating Procedures was a part of the training]. For the longest time, they didn't really have properly written SOPs for their labs, and even the few that they did have, it was more or less taped to the wall, which could be easily damaged. So today one of them demonstrated their new system developed after the training that works really well, and she showed it to the entire class and everybody just lit up like they were so excited. A bunch of people were scribbling to write down what she was showing them so that they could take it back to their labs to use. So I hope that maybe not Haiti as a whole is going to benefit from the trainings that we're doing, but at least the lab culture, the clinics in Haiti will definitely benefit from it.

This is good evidence that graduates of a previous training were able to implement what they had learned in the Partners in Health facility where they work. It also indicates satisfaction on the part of the trainees, which is confirmed by the results of our post-training assessment. Of nearly one hundred laboratory workers who completed the survey, 93 percent answered "Certainly" to the question "Are the skills you learned this week useful in your laboratory?"

Many trainees indicated they would be able to apply the knowledge they had just gained in the training and said that their new skills would improve the quality and accuracy of their laboratory work. Some even mentioned that the training would give them more confidence in doing their work. Beyond the specific information they learned, other advantages they identified included that they could now teach, share, and lead with this information; that the training was applicable to other aspects of their lives, particularly in managing family, church, and other social groups; and that the training would allow for improved laboratory management.

Unfortunately, fewer than a quarter of trainees could say with certainty that their laboratories had the equipment necessary for them to apply their new knowledge. This raises questions about the sustainability of training when its lessons cannot be implemented.

In addition to formal training and institution building, there are many informal but helpful ways in which volunteers were reported to have passed along their knowledge. A community health worker in Ecuador told my assistant, Joe Rendon, "Last time they came they showed us about first aid training. That helped us a lot because none of us knew about that." A Haitian nurse working in a clinic in Port-au-Prince with Heart to Heart volunteers said, "Sometimes they give us not information but an explanation that is new to us, so it serves as an apprenticeship to a certain extent." Another hospital security officer in Niger insisted, "They bring a lot of things to our hospital: their knowledge; their participation; some train the nurses and the administration."

An ob-gyn physician in Ghana appreciated the willingness of volunteers to adapt their tasks to the needs they saw.

> We've had so many instances where when they come in, they identify some of the problems that we are facing and when they go back they talk to their supervisors, and then they try their best to help with whatever means that they can. For example, these young guys came down here and in trying a machine that we were using for salvaging the blood, they realized that what we were doing wasn't that effective, and most of the time we ended up throwing our blood out. So they researched how they can develop an instrument that we could use to salvage or sieve or filter the blood that we get from the peritoneum and give it back to the patient as a transfusion.

Developing or improving physical infrastructure may be part of capacity building and can also be an important contribution. "Something as simple as rebuilding the clinics, I know that sounds crazy, but that affects the confidence level, right?" said the director of a faith-based NGO. "Someone walks in and sees black mold on the wall, do you think your doctor's going to take care of you? But they come into a nice clinic now that has electricity and running water, a good pharmacy. That improves the confidence level of that doctor and that institution, because that's all people can judge."

Nathan Darity of Amizade cited examples from his organization's work. "It's easy to see the infrastructure changes that are a direct result of volunteer hours," he says. "We built community centers collaboratively with our volunteers and local volunteers. We've built wings of the clinic and the dormitory that houses volunteers at the clinic." But he recognizes that buildings are only a small part.

Improved Patient Well-Being   In attempting to assess the impact of volunteers in health programs, I was constantly asking about evidence of improved health status. Comments about patient improvements most often referred to surgical missions, where the impact is rapid and often dramatic. For instance, a local hospital social worker in Niger told interviewer Susan Rosenfeld, "Sometimes the impact is visible. With surgery especially. When a specialist comes for noma [a disease caused by nutritional insufficiency, in which the faces of people affected are grossly disfigured], the results are really visible. We only do noma operations when the specialists come."

A local nurse in Niger described a volunteer surgeon who comes to repair cleft palates. "He operates on thirty-five children and he resolves a lot of problems. All the operations are successful and the children return to their villages. The children were desperate, without hope. You think that all your life you're going to stay like that. Your age-mates make fun of you. Maybe because of your handicap you don't even go to school."

A host in Ecuador explained, "When someone has a walking defect because of a problem on the hip and they can fix it, they are fixing their life. That is amazing. If you can see one of those patients it's amazing, because they feel their life change."

Volunteers with other medical specialties also may leave some notable evidence of their work. "When we first put the dentists in," explained one organization director, "they were completely overwhelmed. Now it's more regular, which tells me there aren't as many people with dental problems that have been brewing for a long time." The same person also cited the impact of volunteer eye specialists.

Over the last seven years, probably there are 180 people who were blind who aren't blind anymore. D. is a good example. He had had cataracts for twenty-five years. He was fifty. He developed young, abnormal cataracts in both eyes, so for twenty-five years he had been totally dependent on people. He also had diabetes and high blood pressure and was overweight. Dr. John took out the cataract on one eye one year. We came back the next year, he had lost the weight, sugar was normal, blood pressure was normal. He was working as a mechanic now. That's what he had done before he got the cataracts. The next year they took out the second cataract. Now he brings people every year that he finds that are blind.

The evidence for patient improvement is not as dramatic in programs of screening and prevention, but study participants also referred to these sorts of benefits. A community health worker in Ecuador, speaking of preventive care, reported, "Before the brigades started there was more malnutrition, no hygiene, lack of health knowledge, they believed that medications had no effect. Now people see that it is good because of the deworming medication and help for anemia. The majority of people are not as sick and there are fewer deaths. The communities are more aware of diseases, are vaccinated, and are grateful for the visits Timmy makes to marginalized communities."

John Adams, administrative director of PINCC-India, reported a decline in detection of abnormal cervical cells and attributed it to the screening that had been done and the treatments already given in the past.

> The director of the Ashram's mobile hospital just wrote us an annual summary, and he said the number of people coming for screening is still the same, but the number of lesions they're seeing and the number of times they're required to do treatments is beginning to decline, because they seem to have over the last three or four years discovered most of the people that were in serious risk. We're used to seeing 6 percent, one out of 16 needing either cryo or LEEP procedures. [Most recently, they found only] 15 people out of 1,200. That's a big reduction. We're just finishing up our fourth year, and it takes five to ten years to see the population level reduction in the rate of cervical cancer. This is the first indication we've had, this recent report, that it's actually beginning to make a difference.

The effects of surgery and the detection of disease in early stages can have dramatic effects. But how do we know if primary care makes a difference? Staff members reported patient satisfaction as one important indicator. A Haitian interpreter recalled, "Sometimes after the clinic, after they get the medication, they always say, 'You have to translate for me. Please tell the doctor for me that I appreciate the way he works, I appreciate the way the doctor takes off my pain and the medication was really helpful.'"

Sometimes, a single case stands out. In an evening discussion in Ecuador, a volunteer physician told the story of a seven-year-old boy she had seen on an earlier trip.

[He had] an undescended testicle, which makes him at a higher risk for testicular cancer, and we referred him to urology. I recognized him when he walked in today and asked the mom about it. And she very proudly pulled down his little shorts and showed us his little scar. He had a beautiful little scar on his abdomen and everything went really great. Here's testicular cancer that was avoided, and he was identified, even though it was late for our standards at seven years old, but it's just wonderful and here he is coming in with a cold and still doesn't like to see us because he didn't like us then. And I just thought it was great that he has the opportunity to not even like us. It was nice to see the system worked.

Often, the improvements in patient well-being are more general, related simply to the fact that patients who once feared doctors or found it too difficult to get to health care facilities report feeling better. Patients in Ecuador told my student Joe Rendon that Timmy is the first or only clinic they have been to. They come by bus or taxi from as far as an hour away; some even come from the city. Patients say their community has improved. One told Joe, "I felt better after the last visit." This was backed up by one of Timmy's Ecuadorean employees. "With the medication they give, the people say they are healing and getting better. They are happy and satisfied with the medication they bring from the U.S., and it is really important for the community."

Also, from an Ecuadorean who works in one of the communities that received Timmy brigades came this comment: "People are afraid of seeking health care, especially at governmental health centers. These brigades bring medical attention to them and help people get familiarized with it. There is difficulty walking to government health centers. Getting there is a big problem, and with these brigades they lose that fear and timidity. This trust was created because of the way they treat people. It is not 100 percent better, but their health problems are not as bad as they used to be."

In Haiti, people who once had little or no access to health care know a doctor will be available on a regular basis. "Here in this clinic," said a Haitian nun whose convent is located in a remote town and who assists with the Heart to Heart volunteers and staff when they arrive once a week, "we do not have the possibility to pay a doctor, but every Friday we have a doctor from Heart to Heart come to help. It's very good, because in this area we do not have hospitals. If someone is sick, and he wants to go to the hospital, he has to walk like four hours. It's really hard. Now they know every Friday they can get to see a doctor. Every Friday in the morning at 6:00 we have so many people here waiting. It's really helpful because we have less people dying."

A local government official in Ecuador explained, "Without these organizations, some people would have already died. They have been saved from serious illnesses, because our culture is not to go to a hospital, they just wait to die, especially the peasants. [Now] there are people who need surgeries in Quito, and without these foundations who pay all the costs, peasants would be left to die. Foundations such as Timmy give these patients hope for life. In this sense it is very favorable for the country."

It is very important to emphasize that these examples come from programs with a consistent presence in the countries where they work. Many volunteer programs lack this important element of continuity. Not only won't they know about the positive effects of their trip; they will also not be there to discover complications and problems caused by their visit.

Probably least visible is the effect of training of community members around health education and promotion. Becton Dickinson and Heart to Heart International held weeklong sessions for people selected from their communities in rural Haiti to become health promoters, repeating the sessions for three different groups. At the meeting of the Becton Dickinson volunteers in Haiti on the last night of the trip, those who had done the training for community health workers in a remote part of the country noted some evidence of the potential impact of their work. "The people in the countryside were so hungry for information and interested and wanting to use it," one volunteer explained. "They see the utility of it. Evidence of that: at the end of the second week, we graduated the second class out there and we were sitting around talking and two guys from the prior week's class came around and were talking to the second week as a group and telling them, 'We're going to mobilize, we're meeting next week, we're going to mobilize and put this thing in motion.'"

Of course, good intentions do not always turn into change, and usually there is no follow-up to know whether they do. In the case of the Becton Dickinson-Heart to Heart training, though, it was possible to gain some insight into its impact. A year after the training just described, a Becton Dickinson group of volunteers returned to the same location for follow-up training with the same community health workers. Two Lehigh University students accompanied them and reported this feedback from focus groups held the first day of each week: "We did discuss how the returning participants utilized their training from last year, and there was resounding positive feedback that it was useful and enabled them to conduct more home visits, community meetings, and house-to-house info sessions. Some even claimed that fewer people were sick in their community." On the down side, repeat trainees answered the training pretest questions no better than did new students, although they covered some of the same material as in the previous session. Ideally, one would want to assess the actual health and behavior changes in the communities to confirm these reports.

The fact that there was a return trip and follow-up research made it possible to learn, even if indirectly, about the impact of the training. But this does not often occur, and it happened in this case only because I asked the students to inquire about it. There was no other effort to evaluate the effects of prior training.

Nonhealth Benefits to Host Communities

Though all the programs considered in this book aim at improving health, host-country staff members note that they bring other benefits to their countries as well.

Financial and Employment Benefits   Volunteers spend about $1,500 each in program fees, some of which goes to paying expenses in the country they visit. They often also travel and shop in the country. Thus they make contributions to the economy, the tourism industry, and local vendors and to communities more generally. It is not nearly as much as what they spend on airfare, vaccinations, and administrative fees—money that stays mostly in the home country—but some host-community members staff considered it an important contribution.

Barrett Frankel, an American working with volunteers in Rwanda, notes, "Volunteers generally spend some extra time in Rwanda either before or after their time at Agahozo-Shalom, so on a larger scale they are contributing to the tourism industry in Rwanda by trekking with the gorillas, going on a safari at Akagera National Park, spending time in Kigali, or going for a hike in the Nyungwe Rainforest."

Staff members in Niger concur. "It's an advantage for the country," says one of the security staff at the CURE hospital. "At the end of their stay they buy souvenirs, and poor families get something when the volunteers purchase souvenirs from them." As another CURE hospital staff member explains, "Volunteers, when they come, they spend money. There are crafts, artwork; the volunteers like that; they buy that in order to have souvenirs of Africa and of Niger. They look at the giraffes, they take photos, they pay the guides."

Economic benefits can be captured by design. "If it's done right, it's bringing money to an organization, it's bringing money for community initiatives, but it's also bringing money into people's pockets," says Brandon Blache-Cohen of Amizade. "In Jamaica, for example, sixty-five families (who house the volunteers) make an income with each program we run. In Tanzania, a semester program might inject $40,000 or $50,000 into people's pockets. In our programs in Jamaica, 65 percent of the funds that a student will pay end up in the pockets of real people and that has meaning to them."

Quite often, volunteer programs hire local people to assist with arrangements. Says one Haitian clinic administrator, "Some [local] people are working here because of volunteers. If we have no volunteers, there will be no work for the translators. Yes, the presence of the volunteers helps people to continue to work, because that's what they do. No volunteers, no work."

A staff member in Niger, though, describes a possible contrary effect on local employment. "If the fact of having volunteers means that the hospital doesn't need to hire someone, that frees a part of the budget and that helps a lot. The biggest advantage is that we don't spend our money but more work is done." This staff person perceived the savings as a benefit, but it does raise questions about whether more people in Niger might have been employed as staff if the volunteers had not been there.

Feeling of Solidarity with Volunteers   Reports of medical missions often mention solidarity as one of the benefits for host-community members, who get a feeling that "the outside world recognized their plight."[1] This sense of solidarity is confirmed by many host-country staff members who emphasized the importance to their local communities of perceiving that others from the outside care about them. And it is recognizable to the volunteers.

"When we came to a village," says John Adams, "the leaders of the village would come out in the road to do a *puja* on the vehicles, a Hindu holy ritual for welcoming us. They'd sing, they'd smear turmeric powder or other powders on the buses, and just make a big deal out of our arrival. That happens every month." Adams draws a conclusion from this demonstration that may or may not represent the actual feelings of the community members: "They absolutely adore the mobile hospital and they trust us completely."

An Ecuadorean man who works for Timmy and has also assisted other organizations bringing volunteers to his country explains that this is very difficult to measure. But, he says,

> people really feel cared about, and I think that's something really, really nice. Many people, they feel very grateful, because they feel that someone takes care of them. The people there on the Amazon say, "We are not very important for the government." There are racism problems in the country. We don't have a lot of resources for going to the hospital and actually we're not very important for the rest of the country. But when someone comes here and puts in attention, spends their time, spends their resources, you can feel that there's an interest and that's something very valuable. You're actually affecting the life of the person, not only about the current problems, but also about how they face life. People feel grateful, people feel important because of that care.
>
> For example, many of our patients tell us that when they went to the public hospital, sometimes the doctors don't even want to touch them because they're covered with mud, they're sweating, they come from farms. It's the way they live. Most of the doctors study in Quito, and sometimes they come from wealthy families and there's a prejudice behind indigenous people that they are dirty, they are slackers, and things like that. So there's a barrier. I think that's one of the main reasons. And the other is because of the commitment that the majority of the volunteers have about their patients. They're passionate. They are serving with the same attitude as they do in the United States, and people can feel that.

Margaret Perko, a medical student at University of Minnesota, has volunteered many times with the same project in Uganda. "There was one group we worked with," she told me, "and we went to give them the medicine and train them, and it's a long trip, it's an all-day affair when you go there, and it's a stressful day. They were so thankful that I would come back and see them. It was overwhelming because they said, 'Thank you. We know that you love us, and we know that you care about us, because you came back.' I think the idea that we come back every year, and they know we're coming back and they trust that we're going to follow through, gives them a hope that someone cares about them and someone is investing in their future."

It is difficult to know what to make of expressions of gratitude, though these are often cited as evidence of the value of medical missions. Surely the norms of hospitality in many cultures require such expression. It is also the case that volunteers bring financial benefits apart from any impact they may have. Appreciation and gratitude are very satisfying for the volunteer, but they are not proof of valuable accomplishment.

Solidarity is clearly an important dimension of volunteering that may have a big impact, even if it is particularly difficult to measure. It does, though, have the potential to produce disappointment, especially in the modern era of online social media. Barrett Frankel, for instance, worries about volunteers giving out their contact information to people in the host country and then never following through when they get home. "If [the volunteers] agree to be a Facebook friend," she told me by e-mail, "they are committing themselves to staying in touch with the [Rwandan] students for years to come; the same goes for e-mail. I remind them that it's OK to say no if a student asks to exchange e-mails because it is better to be upfront and honest than to lead the students on and let them down in the end, as they have had a lifetime of disappointment and do not need to be disenchanted by volunteers from the Western world." What may seem like an act of solidarity means nothing if it isn't accompanied by a sense of obligation that goes well beyond demonstrating caring for a week.

Social Capital   Another potentially positive aspect of solidarity for host-country communities and staff members is the social capital they may gain by developing connections with people from other countries who may then be able to help them with their personal goals. For example, one Haitian staff member said, "Sometimes, we meet some volunteers who are willing to help us to go to [medical school in the United States]. I expect that they are going to give us more advantages. That's what I thought, that the people of what you call international organizations will give us access to go to another country." It seems clear from the comment that this has so far been an unrealized hope, although there are cases in which a volunteer does help host-country residents gain admission to U.S. schools.

Claire Wendland, the University of Wisconsin anthropologist mentioned in the introduction who worked in Malawi for two decades, also notes the value in increased social capital, asserting that it can produce connections between host-community members and visitors that are lasting and enriching to both.[2] She also observes that interactions with overseas volunteers can have positive benefits for host-country staff identity by virtue of the contrast they offer. Malawian medical students, for example, might recognize in their encounter with volunteers "a vision of Malawian medical practice as hellish" but in doing so may fashion an image of themselves going forward as "more flexible and creative, as more committed and empathetic, and sometimes as better able to see the big picture of health and disease: that is, as practitioners of a better medicine."[3]

Brandon Blache-Cohen of Amizade provided an example of how the presence of a volunteer organization can increase some kinds of advantages for a host community as a whole. "There's another multiplier effect which happens sometimes," he says.

> Their ability to pressure government and other stakeholders around them increases when they have foreigners visiting their communities. So in Jamaica, another good example, we got a school built in this little town that we partnered with. All we had to do was send a letter to the government stating that if they didn't build this school that was desperately needed, we would build it and name it after our site director who they were afraid was going to run for office and beat them essentially. This is no exaggeration: within three months bulldozers and cement trucks started showing up and they built a school.

7

"First, Do No Harm"

The Unintended Negatives for Host Communities

> The myth is that you can show up in a random, rural community and hand
> out antibiotics and actually have an impact on patients. . . . If the best way
> to provide health care to low-income communities was through short-term
> trips, then you and I would be going on short-term trips to get our health
> care. Clearly not the best way to do it.
>
> —Matt MacGregor, Timmy Global Health

Many people involved in the field of volunteering are quite aware of
the possible negative effects of short-term volunteer trips. At a 2012 conference of the International Association of Research on Service Learning
and Community Engagement (IARSLCE), there was a wide-ranging discussion of both positive and negative results for communities when students visit as part of service projects. In addition to the many positives, the
conference-goers had quite a list of negatives. Communities risk becoming
increasingly dependent on outside assistance. Volunteer visits may reinforce existing privilege and power differences in the community by providing additional resources and skills only to *some* members. Volunteers
may deplete local resources and waste precious time of local professionals.
Exposure to unattainable wealth (in the form of expensive items owned
by visitors) may create problems. There may be disappointment over the
lack of impact. Discussants even noted that short-term visits may break up
marriages, presumably as a result of liaisons between volunteers and hosts.[1]

Others who send volunteers also recognize drawbacks. Speaking of Haiti, Rebecca Reichert of FAVACA told me, "You really need to be training Haitians and not just sending people down back and forth, back and forth. You're enriching the airlines, but you're not really accomplishing much long term." Dr. Neal Nathanson of the University of Pennsylvania School of Medicine offered a sobering assessment. "I would say that at best it's neutral. In other words, the cost at best is offset by what [volunteers] may contribute, but I wouldn't want to say that they're a real asset." And a volunteer, asked about the value of the trip, said, "I don't know. I think after this trip I might do more just sending the $1,500 check."

Host-country staff members express less open skepticism when asked about the most difficult part of having volunteers come from other countries. None mentioned the concerns raised at the IARSLCE conference. "There are no disadvantages," a host staff member in Niger told Susan Rosenfeld, an American who has lived in Niger for many years and has worked with several organizations that receive volunteers. "There are only advantages [and] no extra expenses." Even the time required to help volunteers is largely not seen as a negative. Many host-country staff members consider this part of their jobs or believe the advantages outweigh any problems. This was the same in all four countries where staff members were interviewed.

Still, some of them raised concerns. The comments fell into a few main categories: taking extra time or creating more work or inconvenience, extra expense, and uncertainty about the future. Additionally, some staffers believe volunteers simply do not contribute anything worthwhile, which must lead us to question whether the time and money invested are being wasted.

More troubling than the inconveniences is the possibility that volunteers may cause actual physical or economic harm, a concern raised by some critics of the volunteerism enterprise.

Extra Time, Work, and Expense

The most practical problems involve time, attention, and possibly expenditures that may put a strain on communities. These strains are probably invisible to outsiders. After all, most traditional cultures have norms of hospitality that require them to welcome and feed outsiders. When those outsiders offer help and bring gifts—even unwanted gifts—it is also typical to express gratitude. It should not be hard to imagine, then, that volunteers may impose costs on hosts but believe their visit was appreciated.

Volunteers from other countries require a great deal of attention when they first arrive; as we saw earlier, there is almost always a period of initial adaptation to the country and work environment. Some organizations have local workers responsible for arrangements and supervision as part of their jobs, but in other cases these responsibilities must fall to the hospital or clinic staff or to local community leaders.

"It is a lot of work to coordinate the details of [volunteers'] visits," said Leron Lehman, who at the time of my interview was director of the CURE hospital in Niamey, Niger, "to set and manage expectations appropriately and to make sure they are properly cared for during their visit. We organize transportation and meals for them; many times we need to provide interpreters, and they simply have a lot of questions that need to be answered."

Lehman's perspective is fairly typical. A host staff member in Ghana told of occasionally missing the bus home because of having to stay to help out volunteers. Another staff member in Ghana said, "I've not seen the contribution. They only waste our time, especially my time."

Wasted time is a big part of host staff perspectives. For one Haitian, the arrival of big groups can mean having to remain at work for many hours beyond the normal quitting time. From Niger, we heard about the "extra load" caused by volunteers who want to visit places and have to be taken. And "if they have problems, we help them. Problems of their household, of maintenance, etc." Volunteers' expectations for their living conditions sometimes lead to complaints; hosts have to take time to respond. Having to provide interpretation also takes time away from the work of the local staff, as does finding others to interpret. Transportation is another issue raised repeatedly.

It should be noted that comments about time wasting were most typical from Ghanaian staff, who are all employed by a Ghanaian hospital, not an outside volunteer organization. The volunteers are often American graduate students there as part of research projects and thus much more likely to be perceived as distracting from or getting in the way of regular work responsibilities. In Haiti and Ecuador, local staff members interviewed for this study work directly with volunteers to deliver medical services and in some cases are paid by the volunteer organization.

American expatriates living in hosting countries and working with volunteers were among those most likely to cite the intrusiveness and demands on time made by short-term volunteers. Barrett Frankel worked in Rwanda for a youth village.

> It takes a tremendous amount of organization, planning, and preparation to make the Village ready for volunteers. Not only does it require time and effort prior to the arrival of volunteers, but while they are in the Village, much of my time is spent tending to their needs and activities rather than devoting time to the Village itself and its people and activities. It may be interesting to note that the Western full-time residents [who are year-long volunteers or fellows] in the Village see short-term volunteer groups as being intrusive and disruptive. Although the Village makes a small amount of money from the volunteer groups who visit, the amount of work and manpower that goes into managing them seems to be far greater.

Breezie Mitchell, a Peace Corps volunteer in Kenya who worked with short-term volunteers, provided a longer-term perspective.

> The most difficult part about having volunteers come is that the projects they complete are not sustainable at all. They finish projects and feel a sense of accomplishment, but once they leave, the projects crumble to the ground because the host-country nationals didn't understand or don't know how to use what the volunteers introduced. It seems as though these volunteers want to help Kenyans become less dependent on donors, yet since they are here for a short amount of time, they do not completely understand the culture, people, or what the community needs. Thus their efforts are somewhat unsuccessful.

In other words, time wasted during each volunteer group's stay may add up to a lot more time wasted trying to accomplish health-related goals over the long term. On top of that, the lack of continuity imposes a long-term cost (discussed in detail later in this chapter); since many volunteer groups arrive sporadically or visit once or twice and do not return, the investments of time and energy host communities make may often seem wasteful.

Consider the perspective of Sue Rosenfeld, who has worked in Niger for many years.

If the [overseas] church supporting a family or a missionary team wants to send people over here, it is very difficult to say no to them. But it requires a tremendous amount of logistical and sometimes financial support at this end. And it takes the missionaries away from what they are here to do.

These volunteers do not have the language skills needed. So the mission team here has to either translate or organize a team of interpreters. And they have to house these people and they have to feed these people, and for missionaries living in the bush, that can be difficult or almost impossible, if there are picky eaters or people with dietary restrictions in the group.

Rosenfeld further draws a contrast between volunteers who have specific skills and those who don't.

Skilled practitioners—builders, engineers, surgeons—can perform a real service here. Generalists—well-meaning people with no specific skills who come out on short-term mission visits, those who "teach the children to wash their hands" but can only do it in English—are a drain on resources and often come away thinking that they have made a "real difference" when all they have done, in my opinion, is taken a lot of photos, had a "feel good" experience and stretched the resources of the mission here. But if support is contingent on these visits—and sometimes it is—the missionaries know that they have to just "suck it up," smile, translate, answer stupid questions, take people shopping, etc., so that the churches from which these volunteers come continue their support.

Rosenfeld's points are echoed by other expatriates who have spent significant amounts of time in host countries and who have seen many volunteers come and go. Her observations apply to local NGOs and health facilities as well to missions. They belong in any serious calculation of the value of short-term health-related volunteering.

Faculty based in the United States who send students to other countries also recognize how those volunteers can impose on the local staff without necessarily providing an overriding benefit. "The medical students have to use one of the local nurses who's bilingual as a translator, but that takes the nurses away from their regular duties," says Dr. Neal Nathanson, "so yes, they are doing something and they are doing patient care, but I think it would be overly optimistic to say that they're much of an asset. On the other hand, you spend a lot of your time just explaining how the system works, and they get under foot at times."

Dr. Nguyen also has concerns.

If you go to a place where they don't have a system set up already for visiting interns, that can be a great drain on the leadership of the organization in order to provide adequate supervision and education and kind of
hand-holding of these interns as they're arriving and trying to figure everything out. And if the interns aren't there long enough for you to get a return
on that investment, then that's really a problem. Especially now where nonprofits are all struggling just to keep their heads above water to do the work
they already have to do. Now they've got this other set of people here who
need to be educated and they are curious and they want to learn, but they
also have minimal sets of skills, so that can be a challenge.

Sometimes additional work results when many groups want to arrive
in the same place at the same time, challenging the coordination capacity
of the host-country staff. An Ecuadorean physician told me she never says
no, just that she has to "look at the calendar, because the groups already
have a reservation." She described the plethora of groups coming for different reasons: Canadians, French, Germans, and Italians coming to do
ear reconstruction for microtia (a common birth defect in Ecuador), dental
cleaning, and surgeries for cleft palates, hip replacement, knee replacement, club feet, and hip luxation. So the presence of multiple groups is not
always seen as a problem, since it also means an increase in services.

On other occasions, however, the multiplication of volunteer groups
may not seem so beneficial. As an American volunteer nurse who had
worked in several countries on short-term missions recalled, "I feel like we
have been intruding in some instances, and people just kind of welcome us,
say 'Hey, here comes another group, here comes another.' And buses come
and go, you know, and taxis come and go, but the organizer doesn't seem
to mind as long as we don't harm them."

Claire Wendland offers examples from Malawi of fragmentation of
services, even for the same illness, resulting from the multiplication of
programs that each focus on one aspect of medical care. For example, she
writes that

internationally sponsored research projects and foreign NGOs made enclaves for some technologies, pragmatically inaccessible to students and
their patients even though tantalizingly close by. In 2003, viral loads and

CD-4 counts could be measured in the Johns Hopkins research labs, antiretrovirals were available in projects run by Médicins sans Frontieres (MSF) in Thyolo and Chiradzulu, and one kidney dialysis unit existed in Lilongwe for the use of one government official. None of these were available to patients outside the enclaves' boundaries. The priorities of donors, transnational research projects, and politicians could produce a bizarre hodgepodge of resources.[2]

David Citrin observed a comparable situation in a remote district in Nepal, where there were 177 registered NGOs (approximately one for every 270 residents), half of them working in the health sector with no coordination among them.[3]

Occasionally the extra burden on hosts is financial. A Haitian staff member explained that as the volunteers' host "the only difficult aspect is we have to find funds to make sure their stay is comfortable for them." An Ecuadorean municipal official concurred. "There are some foundations that are costly because they ask for transportation, accommodation, and food, but they have no follow-up program." He no longer agrees to assist such groups; the cost is greater than any benefit. But surely not all communities feel empowered to refuse offers of help, even those with questionable value.

A study of perceptions about health volunteers from thirty-five Guatemalan health professionals revealed a sense that logistical details related to short-term volunteer visits take up the time and energy of local staff.[4] One Guatemalan staff member described himself as "half project coordinator and half tour guide," since he was always having to arrange transportation, housing, food, and interpreters for volunteers. As several studies have found, host staff members are most appreciative when volunteer organizations coordinate with them to provide for needs that cannot be met locally, and this in turn creates less concern about wasted time and energy in the host community.

Potential for Medical Harm by Untrained Volunteers

Medical journals have published critiques of volunteerism focused on the potential for medical harm from students performing tasks for which they are neither trained nor licensed. Harm may also result from a lack of continuity and follow-up and when volunteers compete (inadvertently) with and perhaps even undermine local medical systems.

The anthropologist Lauren J. Wallace writes of "evidence that involvement with medical voluntourism can lead pre-medical students to complete, or be tempted to complete, clinical tasks that they are not qualified to undertake." As one medical student volunteer told her, "When I arrived in Uganda, there was no checking of my credentials—the colour of my skin and my nationality stood as my qualification. During my time there, I was asked to give injections, IVs and set broken bones. Explaining my ethical position regarding providing treatment was one of the most difficult things I had to deal with on my trip; standing by those ethical guidelines was even harder."[5]

That particular medical student avoided overstepping bounds. Others may not resist. Two educators advocating for change in medical school electives report that students are often left to "do their best" with little supervision and therefore may "exceed the boundaries of their competence and learn at the expense of their patients."[6] A review of studies of medical missions found several critiques of the possible harm from treatment of patients by untrained and unsupervised volunteers.[7]

In my own research I came across several very troubling stories of students with minimal or no medical training seeing patients and handing out medications—in essence, functioning as the doctor in remote villages. One particularly bad example came to me in a copy of an e-mail an American undergraduate student majoring in global studies sent to her adviser back in the United States from a remote East African village. She explained that she was diagnosing and treating patients who had walked very long distances to the clinic because though nominally supervised by a local nurse, she was often on her own. The student, whose medical knowledge came solely from reading a book on basic care, was the only outsider during a gap between volunteer physicians. She was acutely aware of her lack of knowledge and found herself torn between wanting to help seriously ill patients desperate for help who had come so far and doing nothing because of her great anxiety about making mistakes. Her adviser told her to leave until trained staff became available.

That experience speaks to an untenable situation that poses psychological risks for students and medical danger for patients. It also raises the question of whether an educated and dedicated volunteer with an informative book and access to a few medications is better or worse for patients than no care at all.

Several untrained volunteers told me the facilities in which they worked were so basic in what they offered that it was not difficult to learn quickly which of the limited set of pills to give for which symptoms. Some said it was "cool" to play doctor; others felt they simply couldn't ignore the very real needs of sick people right in front of them. Local staff may also see the presence of volunteers as an opportunity to take a much-needed break. In any case, there's great potential for disaster. In my view, organizations that sponsor volunteers must be responsible and ensure that these kinds of situations do not occur.

Margaret Perko, as a medical student, volunteers frequently in Uganda. A day after her return from a trip, she discussed her work and reflected on reports from her medical school colleagues about their experiences in other countries. "People come back with their stories about how many babies they caught or how many of these really cool things that they've done, and I cringe when I hear it, because I don't think that we should be doing that as students."

These accounts offer a few examples of a phenomenon of great concern to people responsible for global health programs based in medical schools. They help explain the large number of published articles on the subject in the medical literature and development of the WEIGHT guidelines (an acronym for Working Group on Ethics Guidelines for Global Health Training) for volunteering by health profession students and trainees. Standards have also been developed for undergraduates.[8]

Tricia Todd, assistant director of the Health Careers Center at the University of Minnesota, has had to become adamant about preventing students from exceeding their training level, even if host-country staff pressure students to do so. "A colleague from one of our partner locations in an underresourced community commented that 'if there is a need for help, can't the students do something?' I said, 'Well, of course. It depends on what that something is.' If they are carrying towels from here to there, helping in some way that does not require medical training, absolutely yes. They can be helping move people through lines or registering them. The motto we use is, 'If you can't do it here, you shouldn't do it there.'"

Medical Harm Due to a Lack of Continuity

While articles on medical ethics focus on students, experienced professionals can also cause harm. The founder of an organization with regular missions throughout the year has some very specific medical concerns about one-shot trips. "If you're just going in there for a week, you're making things worse, and we have a lot of that in the Dominican Republic. People just come for a week. They hire a Dominican doctor; they go out someplace and hand out a bunch of medicine. I really believe that makes things worse because rebound hypertension is very real. You put somebody on high blood pressure medications and then they run out and they don't fill it again, and they use medications that have been donated by a local pharmacy that you can't find in the country anymore."

In an era that is seeing a great increase in chronic conditions such as diabetes and hypertension in poor countries (the "double burden" described by Abdesslam Boutayeb as representing the high prevalence of both acute infectious and chronic noninfectious disease),[9] one-shot medication distribution, even by trained professionals, can indeed do more harm than good. People with chronic ailments require ongoing monitoring and medication consistency.

Improving health also requires a focus on prevention—addressing the underlying causes that produce illness. Short-term missions treat symptoms, poorly or well, but they emphasize expensive interventions over meeting basic needs that are crucial to health.[10] One of the principles for effective short-term trips discussed later is the need to focus on prevention.

Matt MacGregor of Timmy Global Health concurs that onetime missions create problems for communities as well as for the more established programs.

> There is competition—I guess you could use that word—in the sense that when you go to rural communities sometimes you often see some overlap in terms of, "Oh, there was just a foreign medical team here." That is something that is a huge problem in certain areas, and it's mostly a problem because it normally happens when groups simply run one-off trips, where they've decided they wanted to do something like this, they make a few phone calls and the local government or a local contact says, "Oh, why not,

they can go out into this rural community and we'll set up a connection for them." The problem is that they go, they set up that connection, no one knows if they're going to return, and they kind of mess up the programming of other groups like ourselves or local organizations that are doing more consistent outreach in those communities, because they hand out different types of medicines, they don't take medical histories on people, they don't keep an eye on those medical histories.

Short-term surgical interventions can create comparable problems with lack of continuity. While there may be immediate and dramatic benefits, there are always risks and side effects with surgery, and if a group of surgeons departs right after the operations, there has to be a process in place for follow-up. That is not always the case.

Annie Liflander, an American physician who worked full time in Nicaragua, is very concerned about this situation. "I observed problems with orthopedics groups who came and went," she said in a telephone interview. "Who was going to do follow-up with patients who had complications? Whose patient was it? These were sometimes bad experiences. Can the local infrastructure support follow-up? What do they leave behind in terms of supporting local infrastructure?"

Dr. Marc Levitt, a surgeon at Cincinnati Children's Hospital, has participated in and led surgical trips to other countries—and has witnessed the same problem. "Surgical missions in general do not go well—there is a lot of effort without a lot of follow-through, not a lot of sustainability. There is a lack of understanding of what is needed on the ground. Teams go and don't know if they make a difference."[11]

This is similar to Linda Polman's critique in *The Crisis Caravan*.[12] The lack of coordination with local professionals is sometimes understandable, such as when no one is available with the necessary training or when needed facilities simply do not exist. But in those cases, performing surgery during a brief visit is probably a bad idea. Programs that do short-term surgical trips are best when they both coordinate with local institutions for follow-up and train host-country physicians to perform the surgery themselves. "The single most important factor before departure from a successful surgical mission site is arranging the follow-up physicians to provide aftercare, should it be needed," writes one group of researchers. "Although it is preferable to return to the same locations several times per year to provide continuity of care, this is not always possible. A well-trained local physician is invaluable. This person should be given contact information . . . to use for post-operative questions."[13]

Maya Roberts, a nutritional researcher, describes a short-term medical trip in which young and untrained volunteers distributed bottles of children's multivitamins they had brought in their duffle bags. That might seem innocuous, but her analysis reveals a variety of ways in which what she calls "duffle bag medicine," if inconsistent with local practices or not integrated into a continuous form of care, could actually cause severe harm to local children. For example, told the vitamins will make their children strong and healthy, parents may rely on them as a future cure for a child's parasites and not purchase more expensive, needed medication. Or the children may take many vitamins at once and become constipated, adding to discomfort from the parasites.[14] That is but one example of how the lack of continuity can result in volunteers' actually causing unintended harm.

A different kind of problem is the anxiety among organizations' in-country staff members about their future. The experience of one-shot mission trips is so common that even employees of continuous programs worry. "Nobody knows that Heart to Heart is going to stay [for] a long-time project," a Haitian host staff member said. "Imagine if the plan changes—they say 'OK, we're not going to stay anymore, it's impossible for us to stay anymore,' so that means everybody will be unemployed." A staff member of the CURE hospital in Niger expressed the same concern "that they are not here permanently. Maybe they leave us right when we need them the most."

Competition between Foreign and Local Doctors

The lack of coordination with locally run services has other unanticipated and potentially harmful consequences. Representatives of organizations that sponsor volunteers were more likely than the host-country staff to raise the difficult question of how they relate to local services and medical professionals. This issue does not necessarily arise when they bring specialty services not available in the host countries or when they provide supplements to existing services. But when they displace local professionals by offering less expensive (or free) services or services patients prefer, this can have profound implications for care.

The impact was seen quite dramatically after Haiti's 2010 earthquake, when hundreds of outside NGOs arrived and set up free medical services. While these services were obviously needed, Haitian physicians in private practice could not compete, and many had to leave the country or find jobs with the outsiders, which often turned out to be temporary when the outside groups left after a few months.[15]

One Haitian physician who now works for a U.S. NGO described the situation faced when one of the Doctors Without Borders programs closed. "All the employees had to find something else, somewhere else to go. And also the population in that area, they had a clinic there they could go to, and some doctors and nurses and medical staff were there to take care of them, but now they don't have that, so it's not too good when you come. Also, when they go to those areas, they establish a clinic, and the private doctors, the ones who are in private business, they had to leave. They had to leave even the area and go to the United States or somewhere else."

A Guatemalan physician expressed concern to researchers that if patients who can afford to pay for their own private care receive free services from foreign volunteer groups, those volunteer groups end up competing for patients with the private Guatemalan physicians (who could perform the same surgeries, but for a fee). He suggested to the North American volunteer group that it perform a financial evaluation of all patients in order to help target those who truly cannot afford to pay for surgery, but the North Americans, noted the researchers, seem to assume that all Guatemalans are poor and therefore do not want to ask about ability to pay for services. The Guatemalan doctor was concerned that the aid provided by volunteers might not actually be reaching the poorest people in Guatemala.[16]

There are several challenging dimensions to this competition. One is that patients, reportedly, sometimes prefer the outside physicians, not only for the financial advantage but also because they may be perceived as being more accessible or more caring. A Haitian staff member commented, "[The Americans] are more polite with them than the Haitian physicians." I heard similar comments in Ecuador, that patients in the Amazon felt more welcomed by outside health professionals than by those who come from the urban elite of their own country and may be prejudiced against the native people of the rural areas.

A Guatemalan surgeon noted that racial prejudice on the part of patients might play a role in this preference: "Guatemalan patients, especially those with less education, tend to put more faith in a blond-haired, blue-eyed, white-skinned foreign physician than their own Guatemalan physicians."[17] This prejudice, the assumption of European and American superiority, is unfortunately widespread and rooted in centuries of colonial and neocolonial influences. It can have a pernicious effect on the relationship between volunteers and host communities.[18]

An expatriate working with volunteers agreed that racism might be a factor, "Volunteers get along well with the patients. The patients respect the volunteers more [than they respect] the local personnel. I wonder why. Could it be because they are white? I don't know."

A Guatemalan physician also noted his resentment of the imbalance in power between outsiders and Guatemalans: "These foreigners show up with their shiny new equipment and do their free surgeries without ever working with any of [the Guatemalan physicians]. U.S. doctors come to Guatemala and practice medicine when and where they want. Guatemalan doctors may have a hard time even entering the U.S., let alone being able to practice medicine there. U.S. physicians are not superior to Guatemalans. I am perfectly capable of taking care of my own people."[19]

The preference for the foreign doctors certainly has a financial aspect. "The brigades diagnose and give full treatment," said another Ecuadorean staff member who works with the volunteers, "while [the state-sponsored health clinics] instead give a prescription and the patients have to wait to get the money to buy medicines."

A third Ecuadorean staff member acknowledged the problem, expressing a desire for change. "I believe the people here keep believing the foreigners do the job better, but the people here now have to take their role and responsibility. It is time for Ecuadoreans to see they can do it."

Two expatriate staff members who worked full-time in host countries commented on the same problem. "[Local doctors are] not a huge fan of any programming," one told me, "because we generate complaints for them. Patients will come get our treatment and then go back to the public system and say, 'Well, the gringos did this and this and this and this, and you did not.'"

Local physicians may find better-paying and more attractive positions with the international volunteer organizations, leaving the public sector and creating broader problems for the host country. Their experiences working with the NGOs may also create more opportunities to leave the country altogether and practice in a wealthier country. As one American who had worked with the World Health Organization in several African countries noted, "The ex-pat doctor's cook makes more than the locally paid physician. Of course that is going to cause problems!"

Most volunteers, as well as many organizers, are surely unaware of these dynamics when they exist. But organizers should be alert to ways in which their insertion into a community can create or exacerbate social class and racial divisions as well as have adverse effects on the livelihoods of their hosts. And volunteers should be better prepared in advance to understand the potential implications of their privileged background when they encounter people with much less power and fewer financial resources.

The problem with competition extends beyond health professionals. Untrained volunteers who spend their time building and painting and providing maintenance services may be replacing local people who could be paid to do the same work.

Finally, and perhaps most important in the context of an overall critique of development aid, outside healthcare services may be competing with the services and priorities of national governments. As the authors of the Code of Conduct referenced in chapter 1 write,

> International NGOs often promote pet projects with idiosyncratic accounting systems, individual reporting systems, and objectives distinct from those of ministries of health. These create enormous management burdens for local health officials. Disruptive turf wars sometimes erupt between competing NGOs as they vie for access to specific geographic or health domains, requiring mediation by local authorities. Many ministry of health officials find it impossible to refuse desperately needed resources, even when they are channeled to NGO projects and away from national priorities.[20]

Of course, many national governments around the world lack healthcare resources and infrastructure and often the will to provide adequate care, so competing with their services and priorities may benefit many communities in significant ways. These are indeed complicated waters to navigate effectively, but sending organizations need to be very conscious of how they enter into an existing system and how they may cause problems in the course of trying to help.

Harming the Communities They Aim to Help?

In his book on short-term volunteering, *When Healthcare Hurts*, Greg Seager lists the following five ways volunteers might harm the very communities they are trying to help because they lack understanding (2012, 252):

1. Without understanding how to maintain patient safety in short-term global health projects, there is great potential for causing actual physical harm to patients.
2. Without knowledge, short-term global health projects often diminish confidence in the local healthcare system and its providers.
3. Without knowledge, short-term global health projects are often paternalistic in nature, offering relief where the only applicable intervention is development.
4. Without knowledge, short-term global health projects often cause economic harm to providers and health systems.
5. Without understanding, short-term global health projects are often more about the volunteers than the recipients of care.

The negative effects of volunteer visits are a serious concern and certainly factor into any effort to measure the real value of short-term health-related volunteering. Visitors who impose on the time of their hosts may make no real contribution; worse, they may leave behind staff and patients disappointed by unmet expectations, patients with complications, expired medications, and host-country professionals deprived of their staff and patients, even their livelihoods.

Over the longer term, the potential for harm lies also in the perpetu-ation of dependency and the reinforcement of stereotypes and highly unequal power relationships among countries. Additionally, there is the major issue of opportunity costs: so many public and private charitable dollars, in the billions of dollars, supporting efforts that may be of questionable value. Those who wonder about the direct costs of brief volunteer trips also sometimes ask whether this money might have produced much greater benefit if spent in other ways. But the stakes in the current system, for organizations and volunteers, make it unlikely that the same monies would be available to spend otherwise.

Part IV

Principles for Maximizing the Benefits of Volunteer Health Trips

We're trying to get away from the term "best practices" and go with "inspiring practices" because best is not best for all.

—Sarah Hayes, director, Global Corporate Volunteer Council

The burgeoning academic field of global health can draw on many reports in creating guidelines for practice. For example, in a 2012 report on maternal mortality, leading international organizations refer to the U.N. secretary-general's global strategy for women's and children's health, which includes "key pillars" for achieving reductions in child mortality and improvements in maternal health: "(i) country-led health plans; (ii) a comprehensive, integrated package of essential interventions and services; (iii) integrated care; (iv) health-systems strengthening; (v) health workforce capacity building; and (vi) coordinated research and innovation."[1] These components are crucial for any health program to succeed in the long term.

A somewhat different but related list emerges from the Global Health Delivery Project at Harvard University, which identifies four main principles to guide the delivery of global health services: "adapting to local context, constructing a care delivery value chain, leveraging shared delivery infrastructure, and improving both health delivery and economic development."[2]

The Irish Association of Development Workers and Volunteers (Comhlamh) has a set of eleven principles specifically intended to guide best practices in volunteering, but almost all of them are focused on providing appropriate recruitment and support of volunteers.[3]

Whether six pillars or four or eleven principles, it does help to have a set of standards to guide global health efforts toward the best possible outcomes. This is certainly true for programs that incorporate tens of thousands of volunteers annually. On the basis of my research and that of others, I recommend nine practices, described in the next three chapters, that would be most likely to have an impact in creating effective health-related volunteer programs:

- Foster *mutuality* between sponsor organizations and host-country partners at every stage.
- Maintain *continuity* of programming.
- Conduct substantive needs *assessment*, with host-community involvement.
- *Evaluate* process and outcomes and incorporate the results into improvements.
- Focus on *prevention*.
- *Integrate* diverse types of health services.
- Build local *capacity*.
- Strengthen volunteer *preparation*.
- Have volunteers stay *longer*.

Of course, not all programs can adopt every one of these principles. For example, prevention and integration of services are more pertinent to those providing primary care and screening than to groups that focus on surgical intervention or training. But the research convinces me that every group considering or already engaged in international medical missions must give very careful consideration to achieving as many of these principles as possible.

Though they may not be "inspiring" (to quote Sarah Hayes) per se, and though some may be difficult to follow, they are certainly necessary if we are to invest resources of time, money, energy, and commitment wisely and effectively for the benefit of hosts and volunteers alike.

8

MUTUALITY AND CONTINUITY

Two Pillars of Effective Programs

Host-country staff members reflected thoughtfully on how programs contribute to their countries and what they think would be the best use of volunteers to meet their countries' needs. They had a lot to say about what makes for the best and worst volunteer programs. Two qualities emerged as essential characteristics of volunteer programs if they are to have a positive impact: *mutuality* and *continuity*.

Principle 1: Foster *Mutuality* between Sponsor Organizations and Host-Country Partners at Every Stage

Mutuality is a concept that comes up frequently in writings about volunteerism. Nadia De Leon, a noted figure in service learning, calls it "deep reciprocity" that is based on "solidarity among equals. . . . The knowledge and expertise of the community members and partners must be valued and appreciated as indispensable."[1] D'Arlach and colleagues, in describing the development of a service learning project, credit the inspiration for their focus on mutuality to the Brazilian educator and philosopher Paulo Freire, who writes in the famous 1970 book *Pedagogy of the Oppressed* of a critical consciousness that is essential for achieving change. In this view, "the concientizado [the person who has such a consciousness] recognizes his or her place, and contribution, in the struggle for liberation. The oppressed concientizado stops expecting that the solution comes from the oppressors and works toward resolving the problem. And the oppressor concientizado listens to the wisdom in the oppressed, rather than ignoring their voice or imposing what he/she thinks is the solution."[2]

In recent years, service-learning scholars have advocated for university-community partnerships that view the community as possessing knowledge and assets, such that the university and community can work together to cocreate solutions to social problems.[3] This is very much in contrast with the attitude of superiority that so often pervades faculty and student approaches to community problems. It is, though, in sync with the view expressed by many of the host-country staff members about foreign volunteers. They commented often about the central importance of volunteers' respecting their hosts and the need for mutual learning.

Christian Kraeker and Clare Chandler found a similar theme in their interviews with Namibian physicians. As one said, "It's very good for people to come and see how people do with limited resources and still provide quite a reasonable job. It's often for somebody who comes out of a sheltered employment setting like you guys, you come into the real world and you see that we're doing similar stuff with similar results with much less resources. If colleagues of yours come to visit for a little while and see how we do things, we learn from them, they learn from us."[4]

The theme of mutual learning stood out in interviews and conversations: volunteers are very welcome and appreciated when the interaction is mutual, when each party can learn from and teach the other. People who have lived their lives and practiced their professions in the host country know they have much to teach the visitors. Volunteers who arrive thinking they have all the answers, that they have nothing to learn, and that others should do things the way they are done in the United States are not appreciated. Fortunately, such volunteers, according to host-country staff members, are in the minority.

My field notes from Haiti reveal the importance of mutuality. "The clinic staff emphasized that it is best when the Haitians learn from the volunteers and vice versa, when it is more of a professional collaboration than a one-way process. They are clearly proud of their professional training and accomplishments and of their work and feel encouraged when visitors praise the way they are doing things."

Staff members in the host countries often realize, as Wendland found in working with medical students in Malawi, that they offer others a model of how to address medical needs creatively when resources are scarce.[5] As a hospital employee in Ghana said, "Volunteers can help. The word is help, not do. It is up to us to do but they can help. So when you collaborate, health outcomes will be improved in Ghana." Further, "I think outsiders would always play a supplementary role. I don't think that they're makers of changing our health system."

When mutuality does not exist, the results are less satisfactory. As a Haitian physician noted,

> Haiti is a Third World country and the United States is a well-known, developed country, so if we're trying to do things the way you're doing in the States, it will not fit here in Haiti. You can come with ideas. We are glad to hear what you think and from what you're telling us, we will decide what can fit in our clinic. When the volunteers come, they need to know that we are all a team; whether they come for one or two weeks, we're all a team. *We* know what's going on and when you come to help, we appreciate that, but please follow what we're telling you to do which is very important. Because we know better how things go here.

A lack of mutuality can be seen not only in some volunteers' attitudes toward how things are done but also in the ways organizations may relate to the host-country staff. Some staff members in both Haiti and Ecuador expressed concern that they were excluded by the organization from having a more integrated role with the volunteer programs. In Haiti, for example, one staff person told about initially being promised "access" but then never being invited to meetings at the volunteer center and never finding out what the "access" amounted to. Another was concerned that his expected work schedule was often ignored, so that any plans to go to school after work could not be fulfilled since he was often expected to stay late without notice.

In Ecuador, the local community health workers and other staff members who worked with us in the clinics did not seem to be treated as an integral part of the health care team. There was no introduction to the volunteers as a whole. At day's end, an American staff member asked one of the Ecuadoreans to take a photo of "the team," but the photo included no Ecuadoreans—a very clear, if unspoken, statement that they were not considered team members.

Ecuadorean community workers spoke at times of their sense of being excluded. "Lately, there is not much interaction with the volunteers because we have not had the time to do it," said one. ""Before, for example, there were gatherings for the *promotores* and the community leaders, asking about how their communities are. The students that came would ask them questions that they would like to know about. But now there is none of that going on. I feel like we need to seek more of a level of community. Lately there has been no attempt to get closer to the community because they are focused on attending more patients."

A hospital employee in Ghana reflected on how people like him who were lower in the hierarchy were not consulted about the volunteers' activities. "When you are doing something for someone it motivates you. It gives you enthusiam to do the work. But when I do [extra] work and I don't get anything from you, I become lazy. So when they come they should not give the money to the top, they should come down and look at people who are doing the work and respect them and do what is necessary accordingly."

Achieving mutuality is one of the many challenges sponsoring organizations must try to address. Host-community members want more than helpful visitors with skills and resources, although these are valuable and greatly appreciated. They want to be involved in the work programs undertaken by volunteer organizations, and they want to be respected. They want a relationship of equality in which each partner learns from and benefits from the other.

Mutuality is difficult, even in a program that has it as an explicit goal. Brandon Blache-Cohen, executive director of Amizade, recounted to me what a Jamaican community leader had said: "I have to be honest with you; this is an amazing partnership for our community. Hundreds of thousands of dollars have been injected into our community in the last ten years, but we don't have any professional development opportunities out of this. We know that your students are going back, putting on their résumés that they worked in a community in Jamaica, but what are we going to put on our résumés? 'Hung out with white people for three or four weeks?' It's not going to get us a job. It's not going to help us move forward."

Mutuality, perhaps paradoxically, means that all those nonaltruistic motivations mentioned in chapter 4—desire for adventure, résumé building, gaining experience, feeling good about oneself—are not necessarily bad things in the context of volunteer trips. Host-community members who seek mutuality seem happy for volunteers to gain from their experiences; that means hosts are offering something of great value. A crucial point here, though, is often missed: mutuality means that volunteers recognize and honor the gifts they are receiving and respect the givers, just as they hope the gifts they bring will be valued. It means an ongoing relationship of respect, collaboration, and exchange, if not with individual volunteers, at least with the representatives of the organizations.

The idea of mutuality directly challenges the hierarchical standard in foreign aid, including volunteer trips, that presupposes the superiority of aid "providers" over "recipients" or "beneficiaries". Eliminating this type of language from volunteer programs is strongly recommended, especially as we know that volunteers do not always provide something useful and hosts do not always benefit. Naming each party as a partner, as volunteers and hosts, promotes a different way of thinking about the relationship that can enhance mutuality.

Volunteer programs, to succeed—indeed, to begin to achieve mutuality—require a partnership between the organization sending volunteers and a local host community or organization. Effective partnerships depend on three main components: responsible partners on both ends, basic agreement on the goals of the volunteer trips, and good coordination. A productive partnership may connect a multinational corporation headquartered in New Jersey, an NGO based in Kansas, and Ministry of Health officials in Haiti, as in the example of Becton Dickinson laboratory training described in earlier chapters. It may link an NGO in Indianapolis with religious hospitals founded by European missionaries and local government offices, as in the case of Timmy Global Health in Ecuador. In some cases, the organization based in the wealthier country owns and/or runs the partner organization in the poorer country. For example, CURE manages its own hospitals rather than partnering with independent hospitals. Or the partnership may be an informal arrangement between two pastors or two doctors or between a student and a school or community organization.

However, almost half of organizers do not always have a local partner.[6] Given the complexity of running a volunteer trip and the potential for mismatch between the sending organization's goals, the volunteers' capabilities, and the host community's needs, this is quite concerning. It would be especially difficult for an organization to know that it is doing something valuable for a host community when there is no local partner to help define the best use of resources and to provide feedback after a trip. The idea that a group of foreigners can "parachute" into another country and decide what to do and how to do it without working with people in the community would surely be intolerable in wealthy countries and should be unacceptable anywhere else.

Organizations that depend on an in-country partnership to define and carry out their missions work hard to develop relationships that make their presence more productive. The challenges, and the importance, are well described by a medical mission organizer:

> The first step in forming any sort of partnership is as much as possible listening to the local community, listening to local leaders, listening to the needs of your partners. The building of relationships is fundamental to building a healthy partnership. So we've spent the past 18 months building our relationships before we developed this plan. And I think that those 18 months are really what's going to make us successful over the next four years.
>
> As large organizations from the U.S., we can go in and push an agenda and throw down some money on the table, and any organization is going to jump to collaborate. But I think that a sign of a good relationship is when someone says, "Wait a second. That's not exactly what we're trying to do." We've allowed space for that pushback so that we can have some real fruitful conversations about what is realistic.[7]

"You need a very strong host," says Dr. Marc Levitt, who leads the Colorectal Team Overseas based at Cincinnati Children's Hospital that has carried out pediatric colorectal surgical repairs and trained local surgeons in the techniques in Latin America and Africa. "The host needs to know what is needed to set up, so there is not a lot of wasted time. [It must be] someone you can correspond with and not show up and patients are not ready. It's an incredible ordeal to get the team organized and if it's not ready, you've wasted time. Almost always, the partner is someone I have met or who has come to Cincinnati for training."

Amizade brings someone from the host community directly onto the team. "In every single community we work with, we hire a local site director," says Brandon Blache-Cohen. "In Jamaica and Trinidad they're actually elder statesmen or stateswomen who also happen to be founders of community organizations, so they're considered staff of Amizade and they help us run all the programs."

Many organizations confront challenges in their relationships with host-country governments. Partnerships with governments can be difficult for many reasons, including elaborate rules and red tape and the need to have personal connections with decision makers in order to get things done. So groups often (though not always) choose to avoid such contacts, though that is not always possible. As an Ecuadorean staff member of Timmy Global Health explains,

> This government became way more strict in terms of permissions and control for the medical brigades, and in general for NGOs because actually there was some corruption, especially in the '90s, and also because this government is very interested in standards. So for example, all the medical missions are obligated to present their list of medicines they are bringing and they are obligated to demonstrate that they aren't bringing expired medicine, which happened in the past. This government has the reputation in the country for being very obsessed with the control about NGOs. It became a little bit rough for moments, but it wasn't impossible to work.

Josh Jakobitz, Heart to Heart International's in-country operations officer in Haiti, describes the process his organization went through to gain government approval, which although not required was believed to be beneficial. "It was about sustainability and what we needed to do in order to be recognized by the government," he explains, "and the government says you can only use these types of people, qualified by these certain degrees, in clinical settings. As long as you are in good standing with the government, you can have certain privileges in the country such as not paying tax on a car, such as being able to buy an unlimited quantity of medical supplies at a high discount. It's basically a right to work. We have easier access to the ministries and government resources. It was about twenty months of work—paperwork, documentation, presentations, lawyers, papers, proof, translations."

A faith-based organization that provides primary care services in Haiti and the Dominican Republic has also opted to collaborate with the government. Says the director,

We chose a different model than most missionaries. Everybody was going around the government. We decided not to do that. We work with the Minister of Health very closely. We have the option of doing our surgical outreaches in private hospitals if we want to, but we've chosen not to do that. What we did was, we kind of said, "What are your goals?" And then what we did was we filled in the holes around those goals. Everything we do we're partnering with Dominicans, we're not overrunning them. If they don't need the services, we don't bring them in.

The director went on to explain that the organization brings gynecological surgeons to the country every year or two, but since its main clinic partner already has such surgeons, she takes them to another province that does not have its own capacity to perform this type of surgery.

One model for partnership, adopted by Amizade, is called "Fair Trade Learning"; it offers local community members an opportunity for professional development and for decision making in the design of programs.

Fair Trade Learning

The organization Amizade has developed an intriguing model, "Fair Trade Learning," for achieving the goals of mutuality and continuity. It "recognizes that the individuals and communities that host students and volunteers are uniquely impacted by visitors and should be offered fair working conditions and compensation, hold significant voice in the orchestration of programming, and be offered proper professional development opportunities" (amizade.org/about/fair-trade-learning/; see also Hartman and Chaire 2014).

Brandon Blache-Cohen explains that "the term came from a staff meeting we had, when we held up some fair trade coffee and we said, is there a way to make learning fair trade? Is there a way we can make our programs be respectful of our communities and show proper voice and let them sort of dictate the way things are run and let them sort of dictate the market value as well?"

Fair Trade Learning aims to put the host community at the forefront of programs. "What we're normally looking for," Blache-

Cohen continues, "is an understanding that our community partners are really running the show. Ideally, our partnerships are going to look like they look in Jamaica, which is a place where we work with a 'housemother collective.' The women get paid a certain amount each day to host volunteers, but then to sort of guarantee buy-in, they're asked to reinvest 10 to 25 percent of those funds that they're making back into a community pot. They then vote on how to utilize those funds, and the community volunteers to increase and improve initiatives in their community."

Nathan Darity of Amizade explains how the model works in Brazil, where a commission of local medical professionals discusses and approves potential programs. In the location where Amizade has been working, there is a program to foster the involvement of Brazilian students. "One really great way to achieve Fair Trade Learning is that we leverage the program fees for every student that we bring into the community," Darity says. "We use the fees to help make it possible for local medical students and nursing students who would probably not otherwise be able to participate, to give them the opportunity to have access to a medical team they would not otherwise have."

"By calling it Fair Trade Learning," says Darity, ". . . we can say, OK, are we actually opening up educational opportunities for people in the community to audit the courses that our visiting professors are conducting? Are we creating opportunities for professional development, and are people exercising new levels of leadership? Are we finding ways to spread the budget that accompanies any group? How well is that money being distributed in a way that's being dictated by our community partners?"

Principle 2: Maintain *Continuity* of Programming

"When an organization is constant, it best serves the community," said a host in Ecuador. As a clinic employee in Haiti noted, "A lot of them come and help for a moment. But afterwards, nothing."

In both instances, they are speaking of the second essential characteristic of the strongest programs: *continuity*, a prerequisite to what is typically referred to as "sustainability." A program is valuable if it is predictable, if the results last beyond the initial visit or period of time, or if it contributes to strengthening local institutions that can continue to provide services into the future.

Continuity does not necessarily mean that an organization will send a steady stream of new volunteers forever. Surely the goal of those who train local medical professionals in surgical techniques or laboratory procedures is to make themselves unnecessary and therefore not to have to return to the same place continually. For example, a team of pediatric neurosurgeons from the United States carried out three one-week trips to Lima, Peru, where they trained and supplied equipment for Peruvian surgeons. They then reviewed patient records for five years subsequent to their training trips and were able to document the success of the Peruvian surgeons they had worked with in carrying out specialized surgeries independently. Even tracking results over time from a distance can be a valuable form of continuity.[8]

Those who are involved in primary care and health promotion, as well as surgery, in areas that do not have ongoing services should ideally continue their programs or ensure that someone else will. If they or their partners do not return to the same site on a regular basis in a way that is predictable, patients' quality of care is likely to be compromised. Host-country staff members cite continuity as one of the most important characteristics of good programs.

Staff members who work with the organizations I accompanied in Haiti and in Ecuador explained why they have a higher opinion of those organizations than of many of the others they have seen or worked with in their countries. One might expect them to offer especially positive comments about their own partners or employers, but their comments are consistent with critiques of short-term trips. As one staff member in Haiti said, "With other organizations, sometimes the volunteers will arrive, or maybe a specialist will come, and they announce the day when they'll arrive, and it's only one instance. There are a lot of people who come and go. But Heart to Heart is different; it's not at all comparable to the others." And another, also speaking of Heart to Heart, noted, "In the southeast I can say that Heart to Heart is the only organization which has volunteers working each month, every month of the year. There aren't any others. And the name Heart to Heart, everyone knows it in those locations."

In Ecuador, a local staff member said, "Other foundations come, but they only come once a year, see patients, and then leave. Timmy comes every two months, makes referrals to hospitals, and is a big help. The people are very grateful to Timmy." And another Ecuadorian noted,

> We've worked with eight to ten organizations over the course of the past ten years. One of them sends ten groups per year; another sends three. All the rest are more like sometimes yes, sometimes no, every other year, every two years. You can come and serve and fix specific problems, say good-bye and never come back, and probably there's nothing, there's not a big difference in terms of a long period of time, but if you come every two or three months and you're following up your current patients and if you are trying to help people with needs of surgeries and things like that, you are definitely making a difference.

Another of Timmy's Ecuadorian partners agreed on the importance of continuity: "With Timmy I have signed an agreement and they do come every two months," he told me. "With them we know the communities that we will see. The agreement we have signed with them is that they have to have six brigades and we know the communities, the people, the *promotores*. I have a plan with them that is sort of permanent. And this is favorable because they do have a program to follow up on patients."

Americans who work for organizations full-time in the host countries also note the importance of continuity. As one American in-country program director stated, "There are two other NGOs operating in the same area. One is similar to us in having [college] chapters, but it offers no continuity and no interpreters. They show up in a village about twice a year and 'ring the bell' for patients to come, but they aren't expected and sometimes there are more doctors than patients."

Josh Jakobitz, operations officer for Heart to Heart International in Haiti, illustrated some of the medical advantages of continuous services.

> We don't do a hit-and-run sort of clinic," he explained. "We don't see eight hundred patients in a week and then never return to that. We have established clinics, established sites. So when we arrive at an area, I can tell the doctors, "You know, at this place you need to prescribe medicine

for thirty-six days, not thirty, because on thirty we won't quite be back here next month. But if you do thirty-six, they'll make it, even if they screw up the dosage or forget or take too many." And the doctors really appreciate that because it's reassuring that the quality of patient care is going to continue. And the volunteers also get to work with the Haitian medical staff and meet some really highly qualified, dedicated doctors who are there, who can say, "Oh yeah, this person has been in for this before, so yes, she can come back in four weeks and we can check the blood pressure, we can check the diabetes, we can check to see if the drugs are working."

Josh also commented on what he had seen some of the faith-based organizations do. "When they build these new churches, they generally bring a medical team along. But maybe they're in [a particular town] for one week and they're never going to go back to that town again, or for a while. So they're treating all these people, throwing drugs at them, but there's no return, no quality of care management."

Other host-country staffers commented on the importance of continuity and the frequent lack of it in the programs they had observed or been part of. "We don't have volunteers here every month," a staff member in Niger told me. "They do their jobs and they leave and maybe three months go by before other volunteers arrive. It would be better if this were constant."

A Haitian said, "It doesn't really help when a person comes for one or two weeks, a month and then afterwards they haven't established a foundation for continuing their access here. And what they do is just for a period of time and after five, ten years nothing works. It happens. People who I don't know have told me that 'Yes, I came for two weeks' and everyone applauds, but after one month, two months there's nothing left."

One of the other advantages of a continuous or repeating presence is that the organization has the potential to learn from experience and incorporate this learning in order to improve services. I saw an example of this in Becton Dickinson's training of laboratory workers in Haiti. Training took place a few times over several years, and each session built at least in part on previous experiences.

During my visit, there were three weeklong training sessions in three parts of the country. At the end of each week's session, it was possible to introduce some changes for subsequent sessions (the fact that a corporation was providing funds helped make this possible). For example, the trainers noticed during the first session that participants did not want to write notes in the printed manuals they received, so in the subsequent weeks they distributed separate notebooks, which trainees used for note taking. Concerns that appeared in posttraining surveys about the food being served were also addressed for the next group of trainees.

Similarly, but with greater consequences, an evaluation after a surgical mission to Ethiopia identified complications, from mild to severe, in 76 percent of patients with noma following reconstruction surgery. Most of these had to do with problems of wound healing. The study led to many changes in patient management during a similar mission a year later, such as earlier admission and preparation of patients and more systematic attention to wound care after surgery; surgical outcomes were significantly better after this second mission.[9]

A study of tonsillectomies during short-term medical mission trips in Guatemala noted that some members of surgical teams routinely stay a week longer in case there are postsurgical complications, and they require that patients stay within an hour's travel to the hospital for ten days following surgery. The team also trains local surgeons in the management of hemorrhage, a common complication after tonsillectomy.[10] These practices add value to mission trips and are designed to reduce harm.

The more typical experience of regular turnover of volunteers leads to the question of how knowledge gained by one group of volunteers gets transmitted to the next. Even when there is continuity of programs, the change in volunteers every week or every time there is a program poses challenges for delivery of care. One laboratory trainer told me he hoped he could return to Haiti to do training again now that he had learned better over the course of the three weeks how to be a more effective trainer in a specific context. But he may never get that opportunity, and other new people will arrive to begin their learning from scratch. Suggestions and feedback from one group of volunteers may never be used to benefit the next group or the host partner.

Surely it is difficult for the sponsor organization, as for the hosts, to have foreign volunteers coming through for short periods and making suggestions to those who've been doing the work for much longer. This is another indication of why systematic evaluation is so important: continuously reexamining procedures is key to making them as productive and efficient as possible.

The consensus: continuity is essential to good care. However, it is often not part of volunteer programs. Just over half of organizations reported having all their volunteers participating in continuous projects. The others are in programs that occur only when the volunteers are there or that are intended to be finished in one visit.

Some organizations sponsor volunteers both in one-shot and in continuous projects. One participant explained, "We have ongoing projects—healthcare clinics—as well as short-term projects, putting a roof on a house that is completed in one visit." Said another, "It varies country to country and with whom they are partnering. We prefer they serve with a continuously operating project like a clinic, hospital, etc."

Organizations that do not have a continuous or regular presence have great difficulty knowing whether they have made a positive difference or perhaps have even caused harm, as we saw in chapter 7. Very often, programs can have a short-term benefit that then disappears. When the Becton Dickinson volunteers carried out training sessions with traditional birth attendants (TBAs) in northern Ghana, they distributed "birth kits" that included flashlights, latex gloves, and disinfectant, among other supplies. In a follow-up focus group eighteen months later, my student Caroline Kusi learned from the TBAs that while they appreciated the kits, the supplies had run out or broken down, and, without replacements, they were back to practicing the way they had before the training. Continuity was clearly lacking.

Without a plan and the possibility for continuity, billions of dollars of international development aid and global health assistance can be wasted. That is the lesson from generations of failed aid programs, and it explains why the term "sustainability" has become so common. Yet onetime visits from volunteer programs are all too common. They compete with local professionals and programs, bring medications that cannot be renewed and may be harmful, and create expectations for relationships or assistance that cannot be met. Though they may provide some benefits for a short while, they are also likely to cause problems and disappointments. An individual volunteer may be able to travel only once, but that volunteer accomplishes the most by joining a responsible organization with ongoing relationships and a long-term commitment to host-country partners.

Mutuality and continuity are not separate from each other. A continuous program requires a strong partner; a good partnership depends on continuity. Valerie Matron, an American working for Timmy Global Health in Quito, Ecuador, explains that ongoing relationships with partners create continuity and improved quality of care. She believes Timmy's success in Quito is "entirely because of Tierra Nueva," a foundation begun by Padre Carollo, an Italian priest with whom Timmy's founder, Chuck Dietzen, developed a relationship. Two foundation staff members are Matron's "bridge to the communities. They have been going on Timmy brigades for ten years. I think that's why it's managed to stay, because it's not just a hospital, it's a hospital with a mission to serve the neediest of southern Quito. They're so invested that it's not like we came in and we sort of tried to fit ourselves in or anything. I feel like we really grew together in many ways."

Timmy Global Health's main partner in Quito, Padre Carollo Hospital, is a facility established by the Tierra Nueva Foundation. Timmy partners with the hospital both for outreach to Quito neighborhoods where Timmy has primary care brigades and for receiving patients needing specialized care referred by the Timmy staff both in Quito and in the Amazon Basin. Timmy is not the hospital's only international partner; groups of surgeons arrive from other countries and organizations several times each year for specific short-term projects. But Timmy's volunteers come most regularly and have established a long-term relationship with the hospital and its governing foundation.

Even in these circumstances, maintaining an effective partnership has occasionally proved challenging, as observed by people involved on both sides. Timmy's full-time staff members in Ecuador are generally young Americans who stay for a year or two before moving on to other activities or returning to the United States. Each brings a somewhat different set of skills and approaches, and each must spend time getting to know the environment and adjusting to the expectations and experience of Ecuadorian partners. This is not unusual for NGOs that sponsor year-round programs; it is even more problematic for those whose visits are irregular and have no staff based in the host country.

The reality of staffing changes makes mutuality even more important to a program's effectiveness. Host-country staff members told my student Joe Rendon in Ecuador that they not only learn a lot from foreigners but also have valuable knowledge to share—knowledge that could have prevented some of the problems and complications they have seen occur. "We have been working with Timmy for around ten years," one of them said. "This lets us know a lot of things. Some of the new young coordinators come in and start trying to implement their own ideas [which can cause trouble unnecessarily]."

A memorandum of understanding is one tool that can help avoid conflicts over the purpose of volunteer programs and the division of labor among organizations. Such agreements need to be carefully crafted as part of the development of a relationship and reviewed and revised periodically over time in response to new conditions and priorities.

Mutuality and continuity are difficult to achieve. They require a great deal of effort and money but are crucial if organizations are to avoid the pitfalls of short-term visits. They make for the strongest programs involving volunteers.

9

Community-Focused Research

A group of surgeons has written about what they call the "Seven Sins of Humanitarian Medicine." We will look at all of them later in the book, but for now there are two worth citing. Sin number 2 is "Failing to match technology to local needs and abilities," and sin number 6 is "Going where we are not wanted or needed."[1] These two of the seven sins address the all-too-common situation in which volunteers engage in activities that are poorly matched with the actual needs and context of their hosts. As a means of avoiding these sins, research is an essential element of international health volunteering—research in collaboration with community partners in advance to ensure that real needs are being addressed and more research after a program begins to make sure it is achieving the desired results.

Principle 3: Conduct Substantive Needs *Assessment,* with Host Community Involvement

Needs assessment is no simple task. Different groups and political factions may not see eye to eye on what's needed and how to proceed. But a deliberate and structured approach to substantive needs assessment can make programs more valuable and less wasteful and can help enlist the interest and commitment of people who can teach volunteers about their communities and take ownership in the process.

I believe the best approach to substantive needs assessment may well be community-based participatory research (CBPR), which brings researchers and community members together to determine the community's most pressing needs or relevant problems, their possible interconnectedness, and how best to proceed in studying them—from which collaborative projects can be identified.[2] The value of this approach is in helping organizations increase the validity of information collected and improve the efficacy of programs planned while involving the community in ongoing assessment.

When the Syrian American Medical Society sponsored short-term medical trips to refugee camps in Turkey, meetings were held with Turkish Ministry of Health officials to evaluate past medical missions to the camps and assess needs.[3] Conversations with health officials are, of course, an important component of needs assessment, but so too are conversations with community-based organizations and community leaders. This first step in creating a good program illustrates the indispensability of having a host partner.

Heart to Heart International offers an example of how establishing a year-round presence with regular partners makes it possible to address needs identified by host communities. Steve Hower, HHI's director of corporate relations, explains,

> I feel like Heart to Heart is making great strides working closely with the communities to identify the needs, figuring out what they want and developing the long-term plan. In Haiti, our staff works closely with the government, the Ministry of Public Health, the local officials, other organizations, like local peasant associations, to really get into the communities, be part of those communities and understand what their needs and goals are. And it's never about us sitting in our global headquarters in Kansas trying to decide what we should do. It's very much from the community. What are their needs?

Jennifer Farrington, Becton Dickinson's director of corporate social responsibility, worked with HHI to develop projects for the company's volunteers in Haiti. She told me, "I think BD has done a very good job matching our areas of expertise with the needs of our in-country partners, and I think that's important for both to have a fulfilling experience. One of the questions to the nonprofit, whenever we first start a program, is what keeps you up at night, what is it that if you had a wish list, what are some of the things that you need within six months, a year, two years out, and then looking at our resources and seeing how we can help them reach those goals."

Sin number 2, "Failing to match technology to local needs and abilities," can lead to an enormous waste of effort and considerable disappointment. For example, BD volunteers on one of the company's early volunteer service trips to Ghana began a weeklong training program for local nurse-midwives. They quickly discovered that the curriculum was much too elementary for these trained and experienced midwives. They were able to shift gears and modify the program but lost precious time and unfortunately probably conveyed to the host community that they had assumed a very low knowledge level on the part of the local professionals. A CBPR-based needs assessment that more fully engaged the midwives themselves prior to the training could have avoided this problem.

That experience may have contributed to a much better process when BD prepared a training program for laboratory workers in Haiti a few years later. Jennifer Farrington and Paula Kapotes of BD told me that together with HHI officials they held lots of meetings and site visits and had discussions with a variety of groups in Haiti over the phone before any volunteers arrived to do the training. That input was likely critical to the program's effectiveness, as reported by participants and a Ministry of Health official.

An NGO director described the needs assessment she had carried out. "We started with a survey," she explained, "[asking] what were the needs in the community? We went to the education department and the minister of health. We surveyed the Catholic Church, which is a big provider of services there, but they do it in small amounts. We went around, saw what services were already being provided, and then decided on the medical services that were actually needed." While this approach is valuable, even more useful is one in which local communities participate actively in collecting the information and making those decisions.

One challenge in conducting needs assessment is good data; often there are few reliable data sources on the incidence and prevalence of diseases.

Lessons from Ghana

Becton Dickinson employees had volunteered in Ghana twice before when Caroline Kusi, a Ghanaian-born student of mine, joined BD for a final three-week service trip in 2009. They had assisted in several locations with medical care, lab equipment and training, and building housing for families of children being treated for malnutrition. This time, BD nurse educator volunteers would again offer training for traditional birth attendants (TBAs) and skilled midwives, aiming to reduce the high rate of maternal mortality in the northern region by providing TBAs with lessons on infection control and referral of mothers needing more advanced obstetric care. TBAs also received birthing kits with supplies to assist them during home births, and the skilled midwives received lessons on obstetric care.

A 2011 consultant report, "Our Envisioned Future; Assessing the BD Volunteer Service Trip Program: Ghana 2007–2009, Final Report" (prepared for BD by Corporate Citizenship)—while acknowledging the difficulty of knowing the long-term impact—cataloged the activities and contributions made during the trips (the "inputs") and the many "outputs" in terms of people trained, patients seen, and facilities improved. They also reviewed benefits to the company, to its employees, to Lehigh University, and to the NGO partner, Direct Relief International. Relying primarily on the accounts of the volunteers themselves and on the opinions of U.S. corporate and NGO administrators, the consultants concluded BD had had a "profoundly positive effect on the capabilities of the Ghanaian clinics" and a "potential impact" on the lives of more than a quarter million in the regions served by the clinics. The three trips cost BD an estimated $2 million in salaries, administration, expenses, and supplies. The report of a "profoundly positive effect" was good news for BD and a perhaps unsurprising conclusion by their hired consultant, but the evidence for it was inferred from services provided rather than from any actual documentation of impact.

Millions spent, long-term impact unknown. BD is ahead of most organizations in at least asking the question and trying to get answers. Still, Caroline's research provides some clues. She learned that the midwives and TBAs believed the training and supplies they received from BD the previous year had contributed to better infection control, more referrals, and fewer deaths—excellent outcomes. But she also reported that the conditions of the focus groups may have created some compulsion to give positive ratings. Further, the training was not always well matched to the knowledge of the midwives and TBAs. And there were concerns about continuity. BD had no plans to return to Ghana, and the supplies they had brought were already running out.

When Caroline returned in 2011, she met with TBAs who had been to the training in 2009. They described changes in their infection control practices and attributed these to the training. Most used the birthing kit they had received, but many items had run out or were not working. They believed there were fewer deaths "thanks to training and the Grace of God." Midwives agreed the TBAs were referring women more to the hospital and that deaths had decreased. This was confirmed by a communication from the director of the health center in 2013.

Did BD's very costly visit to Ghana make a difference? Can very brief training change behaviors and save lives? Possibly. Surely other changes may have contributed to this outcome. And with such enormous resources, how might better planning and follow-up have contributed to even more lasting outcomes?

Organizations that work regularly in clinics or hospitals often keep records for individual patients, which can be analyzed for population-based data on the most prevalent problems and how they are being addressed. This becomes even more feasible with the advent of electronic medical records (EMRs), such as in Ecuador, where Timmy Global Health has developed an EMR program in collaboration with volunteers from Microsoft that offers "the opportunity to develop a database in service of public health," says one of Timmy's physician volunteers. "There will be information gathered about populations for whom that information never been collected before . . . allow[ing] people to dig deeper into patterns of health and patterns of illness that might lead to other kinds of intervention that wouldn't have happened before. I think that's really powerful."

The capacity to collect and track patient data also helps make it possible to address the next principle—evaluation.

Principle 4: Evaluate Process and Outcomes and Incorporate the Results into Improvements

> I have no numbers, I have no stats, but I am sure that lives have been
> changed from volunteers who came with maybe a pretty self-serving reason
> and left with a whole different perspective.
>
> —STEVE HOWER, HEART TO HEART INTERNATIONAL

Evaluation should be a part of every volunteer program. The results should be the basis of consultations with host communities about ways to improve the programs. This brings the community-based participatory research approach full circle. After all, how do we know whether a volunteer trip has been successful, whatever the criteria for success may be? Given all the concerns and criticisms raised by hosts, volunteers, sending organizations, and researchers, this is a very important question.

Great claims are made about lifelong changes in volunteers' attitudes and behavior and about benefits of volunteer trips for host communities. When I set out on this work, I strongly suspected that genuine, measurable assessment of short-term health-related volunteer trips would be infrequent. I am fully aware of how difficult it is to evaluate social and educational programs, including my own lifelong activity as a college teacher.

What I did not expect was how often the evaluation question seemed to take people by surprise. When I asked, "How do you know if your program is benefiting the host community?" I was struck by how often that was met by a noticeable pause in the conversation, followed by "That is a really good question." The assumption of benefit is so strong that even for many people deeply committed to doing this work, the idea that there should be some kind of formal accounting seemed surprising.

Explanations for the dearth of evaluation are easy to come by. Mark Rosenberg, CEO of the Task Force for Global Health, told me, "People hate to be evaluated. When you talk about small programs, they don't want to assess their impact because they want to believe that they're doing God's work and they're making the world a better place and not be pushed to specifics. On the other hand, sometimes the effects and the benefits are going to be very delayed and won't be necessarily for that same community, so you have much more diffused benefits."

Explicit faith-based rationales for the lack of evaluation are even more direct. As Bruce Steffes and Michelle Steffes wrote in their *Handbook for Short-Term Medical Missionaries*, published by the Association of Baptists for World Evangelism, "You are not in a competition to see X number of patients or do X number of cases. . . . The success of your trip will not be judged by numbers; it will be judged by God."[4]

There are other reasons. Perhaps most daunting to those who want to evaluate their programs is the difficulty of doing it well. Ideally, a good evaluation would demonstrate improved health of community members after a volunteer trip. Communities that receive volunteers should have better health than those that do not. Documenting such effects convincingly requires an enormous investment of expertise, time, and funding and must necessarily take into account myriad other influences.

Finally, organizations have had little motivation to devote resources to evaluation. After all, most people *believe* the work is valuable. Anecdotal reports are so inspiring: volunteers return with stories of great experiences, and most donors are more interested in seeing large numbers of people involved (both as volunteers and as patients) than in documented outcomes. This has long been true of social services in general, which is why it is only recently that the United Way and others have begun to require outcome measures from their grantees. Nevertheless, the question stands. Fortunately there are evaluation models that address the problem of assessing outcomes that might profitably be adapted for short-term volunteer trips.

Existing Evaluation Models

Evaluation research is a well-established field of study in which scholars have been developing and testing methods for assessing a wide variety of programs. In recent years, there has been a growing recognition among all types of nonprofit and community service organizations that they lack evidence for program value. Calls for more and better evaluation have accompanied a widening recognition of the need to shift from enumerating *input* of resources (staff employed, money spent) or *outputs* (number of people who attended a program, educational material distributed) to a focus on *outcomes*—the effect of these activities and investments of time, resources, and money on the behavior and well-being of their intended recipients.

For example, the Peace Corps' own evaluations over more than fifty years of activity have focused primarily on the volunteers' learning and on whether their presence improves attitudes toward Americans. A recent shift to looking at outcomes, though, has meant that the Peace Corps has begun to consider whether the communities that host volunteers actually gain from their presence.[5]

Similarly, evaluations of college student "service learning"—projects that incorporate community-based activities into courses—have traditionally focused almost entirely on the students' activities, performance, and gains. Since the mid-1990s, though, a growing number of scholars and community leaders have advocated for assessment of the value to the community of having students participate in off-campus research or service projects.[6]

Several methods for evaluating outcomes are worth mentioning. The United Way in the United States now requires results-based assessment (RBA) from its grantees. The evaluation guides recommend implementing RBA by bringing together staff, volunteers, and community stakeholders to determine goals, create measurable indicators, and then establish a neighborhood agenda that (ideally) leads to better outcomes for the community.[7]

The United Nations Educational, Scientific and Cultural Organization (UNESCO) takes what it calls a results-based management (RBM) approach, similar to RBA. "Traditionally," writes UNESCO, "the emphasis was on managing inputs and interventions and it has not always been possible to demonstrate the results achieved in a credible way and to the full satisfaction of taxpayers, donors and other stakeholders." RBM, though, "is about choosing a direction and destination first, deciding on the route and intermediary stops required to get there, checking progress against a map and making course adjustments as required in order to realise the desired objectives."[8] The RBM approach calls for clearly identifying expected results for program activities and establishing performance indicators and associated benchmarks to monitor and assess progress toward achieving the expected results.

Relatively recent approaches such as RBA and RBM aim at informing organizations that spend billions of dollars whether the programs they fund have any lasting results.[9] They emphasize community involvement in defining goals and measures, an emphasis central to CBPR needs assessment. In this approach, community members are part of deciding on the metrics for evaluation and aid with data collection. They can help give meaning to the results, leading to discussions about program changes and future collaborative projects that best meet community needs.

Many of the principles being adopted by national and international groups are extremely valuable for evaluating short-term service trips as well, but they are rarely applied.[10] To the extent that follow-up studies of short-term medical trips are published, they focus on the volunteers or on surgical outcomes.[11] More systematic evaluations are few and far between.[12]

Becton Dickinson relied on the London Benchmarking Group's (LBG) model to evaluate its Employee Volunteer Partnership Program in Zambia. The LBG is a network of corporate social investing programs, and the model can be used for evaluating these programs.[13]

One group of physicians and public health specialists who carried out an international service program evaluation described their work in "A Model for Sustainable Short-Term International Medical Trips."[14] The model is based on a program of the Children's Health International Medical Project of Seattle (CHIMPS), involving American pediatricians who partner with an NGO in El Salvador, working with the community to provide sustainable medical care. The evaluation involved periodically reviewing patient data to guide future interventions, as well as tracking yearly data from communities in which CHIMPS worked.

Jesse Maki and Munirih Qualls, then students at Harvard Medical School, noted in their study (conducted with faculty colleagues) the lack of outcomes evaluation in short-term medical missions and developed a comprehensive method that involved surveys of host providers, mission directors, personnel, and patients.[15] This generated data on six factors identified in preliminary research as being of greatest importance: cost, efficiency, impact, preparedness, education, and sustainability. Five organizations in five different countries participated; all had been in the field on a regular basis for at least five years carrying out either medical or surgical trips. Each had access to the online results of its own assessment as well as a comparison with the average for all five groups. This is a promising approach that has apparently not yet been widely adopted, although one group did adapt part of the Maki approach to survey physicians who had served on missions in Syrian refugee camps in Turkey. Their objective was to improve future trips.[16]

Evaluating Programs

I asked sending organizations whether they evaluate their programs and, if they did, to describe the focus of those evaluations. Two-thirds of the organizations said they do a follow-up survey with volunteers after their trips, while only 41 percent evaluate the benefits to communities visited.[17]

The focus on volunteers rather than the communities visited is consistent with the view that providing volunteers with a good experience is a very high priority. But it is also the case that volunteers are easier to survey and that the benefits to the communities may appear to be obvious.

Often, volunteer evaluation is done very informally, although some organizations do attempt it more systematically. Some groups debrief all their volunteers at the end of a trip and after their return home. "We do pre and post evaluations with students," according to Brandon Blache-Cohen of Amizade. "We have two different evaluations for students. One is just seeing what they're getting out of it and what they liked and didn't like, very basic stuff. The other is trying to measure some sort of change in civic engagement, so we have questions like how often do you read the news and what level engagement do you have in politics and things like that."

The evaluation of volunteers' experiences is often based on anecdotal reports, usually soon after they return from the trip but occasionally over a longer term. Sam Wolthuis of American Jewish World Service explains, "Afterwards you hear a lot from them. They look for recommendations in the future, they want to keep in touch, or they end up working here."

In some instances, sponsoring organizations solicit feedback from volunteers during volunteer trips, through informal "reflection" sessions. As one participant wrote, "Basically . . . evaluation happens around the table at night. It is a debriefing and prayer time." Both programs I participated in also had evening discussions to share thoughts. But their purpose was not for evaluation; they were more about developing group process and solidarity.

Some organizations keep e-mail contacts and lists of volunteers with the idea of eventually studying the longer-term effect. Dr. Neal Nathanson of the University of Pennsylvania School of Medicine explained that his school wants to keep in touch to determine whether the goal of creating future leaders in global health has been successful. "What we have done is set up a database to keep track of all the students who are going through the program with the idea that you really won't know until maybe five or ten years after they've graduated what impact this may have had. So we are set up for somebody to come along in the future and do that analysis. Whether we're turning out the future Paul Farmers or Jim Kims [cofounders of Partners in Health and well-known leaders in advocacy for improved health] or whatever, we won't know that for a while."

When sponsors do look at the impact on host communities, the main methods used are feedback from partner organization staff members in the form of interviews, surveys, and anecdotes and informal feedback or anecdotes from the host community. One in five indicated they use the very indirect approach of gathering feedback from volunteers to assess impact on the community, and some organizations referred to religious testimony as their method of evaluation.

Another one in five organizations says it collects statistics on activities carried out. Typically, these refer to the quantification of inputs and outputs—amount of medication donated, number of patients seen, and so on. However, there was no indication of any measurement of the results of those activities in terms of improved health outcomes. Volunteer reports are even less likely to be good indicators of effects on communities, and religious testimony may reflect achievement of religious goals but not the health improvements most organizations say they are trying to achieve.[18]

More than 20 percent of organizational representatives indicated they do no evaluations, although some said it was something they "should do." These data support the impression that there is very little systematic evaluation going on to determine whether short-term volunteering has the positive benefits for the health of poor communities that most sponsors intend.

I also asked representatives of sending organizations in interviews whether and how they assess the value of their programs and how they know if the volunteers make a difference. The answers varied widely, ranging from "We just know" on the basis of anecdotal evidence and observations, to "We don't do that but we should," to a detailed plan for intended studies. A few have carried out occasional analyses of statistics they've gathered, but a systematic evaluation process is rare. Yet for many of them, this was clearly a concern they wanted to address.

Many organizations obtain occasional or regular feedback from their partner's staff after a program's completion or periodically over the course of time. For example, Matt MacGregor of Timmy Global Health told me, "We know from our partner organizations that we've donated money to what they've spent that money on, and in some cases, we've received from them pretty clear metrics of what it actually led to."

In contrast, FAVACA, which places individual consultants in a variety of projects, obtains evaluative information quite irregularly. "Nothing systematic," I was told. "Maybe we should do that, but it is pretty difficult. Usually it's in talking to the partners on a periodic basis where they will say, well, the assistance that Joe Schmoe offered is actually now coming to fruition and those laws are now passed and we're at the point where we need to set up centers, so you know, maybe it's taken a year or two, but you know that they've internalized the recommendations and moved forward."

"I go to the pastor and ask him for feedback [after my church group visits Haiti]," Minister Mable Humphrey told me. "And because we work with the Ministry of Health, they tell me what worked and what didn't."

The volunteer coordinator of one sponsor organization described a continuous form of feedback from the American staff members who work full-time in host countries.

> A lot of it comes from our field staff's feedback. I interface with our field staff and the volunteers, and the people that I'm working with on a daily basis, so there's a lot of success stories that have come out of that. For instance, in one of our programs on site, mostly mothers in the community will come

to health education sessions, but then our coordinator will go into the community and do kind of random check-ins with them and check in on how well they're implementing the lessons they're learning. So like keeping garbage receptacles away from cooking spaces, cooking in a well-aerated area.

Some of the evidence of making a difference may be apparent to volunteers in what they see and hear from community members. For example, a volunteer who trained laboratory workers reported signs of success in the reactions of participants. "As far as the laboratory trainees, the enthusiasm when you're showing them the material, the type of questions they're asking, like they want to learn more, they want more information. By the second day, you're having people ask us, 'Can we please get your e-mail address? How can we contact you? Can you direct us to the right person to talk to?'" Of course, enthusiasm is not the same as change.

Leron Lehman, who was executive director of the CURE hospital in Niger, said about training programs, "We can see the improvement in our staff—work habits, technique, patient interactions, and so on—over time based on the training efforts we have undertaken."

Matt MacGregor, former executive director of Timmy Global Health, offered an example of one way he sees the organization's contributions.

> I'm pretty willing to take the leap of faith that if we treat a patient who's told us five times that they couldn't get their hernia surgery because they could not access services via the local healthcare system, and then we help them get their hernia surgery, even if we don't assess the amount of hernia surgeries we've done relative to the amount that are needed in Ecuador, we're still pretty positive that we've provided a great, value-added service for that one patient. If we then multiply that by seventy patients, we can say, the referral system makes sense and is working.

As Matt acknowledges, even "quantified observation" is largely based on inputs and outputs, not measured outcomes. Yet, as he observed, people working in the field over a period of time do witness plenty of evidence for outcomes. This can be seen also in the comments of an American physician working full-time in Niger, who told us, "Evidence is the number of patients seen, the number of surgeries done, the number of people going home healthy, skills that no one else has at the hospital, and skill transfer to the permanent staff [training local personnel]."

I also asked Greg Hodgson of Centura Health how he knew whether it was effective for his group to send two hundred-plus volunteers a year on overseas mission trips. I wondered whether he had any indicators of their contributions.

> That's a great question, which keeps us all awake at night, wondering how do we really know that this is effective and a good use of resources. In our case, I think some of our determinants are looking at that partner hospital and what progress it's making. We do keep track of our clinical groups that go over, how many surgeries are done, how many outpatients are seen. But over the long term, I don't know that those statistics are as important as how we are helping to build capacity locally for health care in that environment, without having groups like ours needing to come in to do that. I think we can definitely see progress in the administrative and facilities side. I guess all we can do is judge by the number of providers that have gone through some of our programs and the training they've received through that.

Several sending organizations mentioned that at some point a student had reviewed their records and written a report as part of a course project. These were onetime events. Others were planning or already taking a more routinized approach such as hiring a person in the home office with training in evaluation to work part-time on developing measures. Occasionally, outside consultants would be hired to study outcomes, particularly for the volunteers.

A FAVACA representative expressed some needed skepticism about the kinds of evaluation that are often carried out. "You get this beautiful report that says all of the training participants were awed by the training, and they're all going to go home and they're going to employ all the techniques that they learned, and you look at a country and ten years later, you've poured all these billions of dollars into it, and you're like, why don't I see any difference? But this report says everybody was wowed by the work that they had done. So you can say whatever you want in a report, but are people actually doing what they say they're going to do, and are you measuring the right things, does it really make a hill of beans?"

When people who work full-time sponsoring volunteer trips respond to questions about how they know whether volunteers make a difference with "That's a great question," it makes me wonder whether they've actually ever thought about the question. Sometimes, they'd add, "I'd love to see it happen" or "It would be interesting to know." Such answers reflected recognition of the need to evaluate, but that evaluation is outside the scope of what they can do.

I asked Steve Hower of Heart to Heart International how his organization measured value and outcomes. "We've had staff who truly believe that volunteers make a difference," he told me. "It's great, but we've never been able to measure, like you said, the impact. And, again, we can give statistics, how many people went, how many patients did you see, how many people were trained, but there's never been anything about, OK what does that really mean?"

Matt MacGregor of Timmy Global Health told me bluntly, "I haven't come across any organizations that do it systematically. We're really good at output. I can tell you how many patients we've treated; I can tell you how much money we gave away, how many medicines we donated. We're not good at outcomes. We're not good at, OK, medicine turned into x."

"We don't ask," I was told by one sponsoring program administrator. "We used to ask them for a survey. We used to, but we haven't asked for it in about a year. What were we going to do with this information? So it kind of stopped. We've been doing the same thing for two and a half years. Is it a good thing? Yes. Are we helping the people of Haiti? Yes, I believe we are. I know I'm doing something good."

Another organizer agreed that formal evaluation is less useful than the effects that can be observed directly: "I can walk downtown now and I see people with glasses on that didn't have them before. I have little indicators. I don't have big research."

The likely value of each of these approaches to evaluation is quite varied. But none of them actively involves the host community in the way advocated by the CBPR approach. They do not rely on hosts to help develop metrics for success or to collaborate on the research.

Evaluation Challenges

I recognize it is very difficult to do a good evaluation. To do it well in any environment requires a great deal of time, money, and skill. To undertake an evaluation in another country, where cultural and language differences may make even the most well-intentioned evaluation effort insufficiently useful and valid, is even more challenging. In addition, evaluation needs to be done over time, not just concurrent with or right after a program, if lasting changes are to be made from the results. This is almost impossible when an organization does not return to the same location and when patients are widely dispersed.

"We ask for this information once a year," Margaret Perko told me. She began working in Uganda while a medical student at the University of Minnesota. The project she is part of provides medications to orphanages in Uganda and trains staff on their use. It includes research on whether the intervention reduces the number of clinic visits for illness.

Perko explained some of the challenges with carrying out the research dimension. "The problem with that, one, [the questionnaire is] in English, but it's to be administered orally through either an English-speaking person or through a person who speaks Luganda, and a lot of the words in medicine are not actually the same. I work with a Ugandan physician who goes with us on all these trips, and even she can't find the words in Luganda to translate to ask the people some of the questions, so that's kind of been scary."

Brandon Blache-Cohen described a challenge even larger in scope when Amizade, the organization he directs, conducted a community satisfaction survey in the countries to which the group sends volunteers.

> It is just a bear of an experience for us trying to do this responsibly in ten countries at the same time. Every single community has a different way of managing and dealing with this, and how do you determine who's taking it [the survey], who's not taking it? There are a lot of people in the community, and they don't all know who we are. They think of us as those white people who show up seven months out of the year or something. So gauging their interest and their satisfaction and their excitement has been very, very challenging. Many of the people who are able to be a part of this evaluation make money from us. Also, the way that you do surveys in Jamaica is collectively. Everyone talks about the question, they sort of come to a group decision, a group answer and then respond individually, so we've had a lot of really interesting experiences over the course of the last year.

Cultural differences seem to be a very common impediment. "While [our partners' evaluation process] is part of our evaluation of our work," one respondent wrote, "it does not hold substantial weight in our evaluative process. There are many issues, including behavior change and cultural issues, that can affect perceived benefit to the community that are completely out of the control of our organization, and thereby, a bad measure of evaluation of what we do." It is troubling that in this case the community's perceptions of benefit are not considered a good measure for evaluating programs.

A volunteer with a degree and experience in public health explained her approach to evaluation, which takes into account that people who receive services may be reluctant to criticize and consider it rude to express dissatisfaction. In evaluating a program training community health workers, she was able to use her own personal history as someone from a poor country in Latin America to gain greater understanding.

> I did an evaluation on the structure and the format of the training itself, strengths and weaknesses. In this culture, which is very similar to my culture, it's a culture that values relationships and I knew it would have been really difficult for them to tell us, "We didn't like blah blah blah." So we emphasized and emphasized and emphasized that by telling us where we fall short, you're helping us. This has nothing to do with our relationship with you; we will not be hurt. We want to come back and we want to do a better job. I even said, "Promise that you will be truthful to us, you will not hurt our feelings, we need this!" And we just took the time to explain to them and emphasize why it was important that they tell us where we fell short so that the next time they'll have a better training. We conveyed the point that this was for their benefit and it will not hurt us, it will not impact their relationship with us. I knew that would have been a barrier to them telling the truth ahead of time.

The challenge of documenting improvements in health is especially challenging where health status data are sparse and unreliable, especially at the local level. Caroline Kusi, my student at the time, was asked by Becton Dickinson and Direct Relief International to show how their intervention in training traditional birth attendants might have influenced maternal mortality rates in the district of northern Ghana where they had sent volunteers. It seemed very unlikely that a few basic training sessions would have such a profound effect, but since there were no reliable data on maternal mortality for the area, showing this type of change was impossible. Data from the Ministry of Health in Accra and from the district health office were not even similar or from the same years.

Despite these many challenges, some organizations and individuals are nevertheless taking on evaluation. They see it as necessary to improve their programs. For example, Timmy Global Health has been working to develop a set of clearly stated goals and objectives with metrics for tracking how close the group is to achieving them. The first step, identifying goals, is not always as easy as it might appear.

"I looked around," explained Matt MacGregor, "and I said, if you asked a person in Timmy's network, even on our board or in our staff to define what we do and why it's important, everyone would answer slightly differently, so we said, why don't we actually map this out and in a real, clear form say here's what we do, and here's why." The result of these conversations was the development of a "logical framework (log frame)" that identifies the major goals and indicators for each. The categories of goals selected for focus in 2012–13 were referral systems, quality of short-term medical clinics, student engagement, and chronic care management. Matt's explanation is worth quoting at length.

> We picked a bunch of very formal indicators that we're going to be tracking over the course of the next year that are all about patient satisfaction, referral system, proper communication with translators, things that are going to give us a much bigger sense of impact. A good proxy I think would be percentage of patients who consistently return. Most of the time, people are returning to something consistently if they like the product that they're getting.
>
> On our referral system data, we know more or less the percentage of patients that have an identified problem in our clinic that show up at our referral partners. We're going to start to track that systematically, because we really believe that one of the best parts of our programming is this referral system. Most of these patients face barriers to health access that would prevent them from getting those types of services or make it hard for them. If we're at 67 percent, we should shoot for a target of 75 percent, and that should be the way that we measure our success internally as an organization. What we're trying to do now is make it more systematic.
>
> So as we do more research on these individual pieces, we're hoping to pull out one or two of the strongest indicators that would apply to each aspect so that we can create almost a dashboard of, look, 65 percent of patients said they were satisfied with our wait time. Our target this year is to improve it to 75 percent. What do we do? My argument is

that evaluation has nothing to do with 100 percent. It simply has to do with what percentage you're at, and what target you set, and whether you meet that target.

In a follow-up email, Matt added, "Let's find a middle ground—if we can ensure that a high percentage of our referred patients received the service they were referred for and told us they had tried to get care in the local healthcare system previously and could not, then it's reasonable to take a leap of faith that we added value to the local healthcare system."

Brandon Blache-Cohen also discussed the organization's intent to carry out more research beyond the patient satisfaction study already conducted in multiple countries. "I've been mandated by the board of directors to develop a whole slew of different data and try to really look from the community's perspective as to what is working, what is not. In fact, ideally, we're going to do some participatory action research. The communities are going to be designing their own matrix. It's very hard. There are a lot of cultural issues that we're running into with that."

The data that sending organizations gather through reports, anecdotes, and volunteer feedback, as described above, tell only a small part of the overall story of how short-term health-related volunteering affects communities. What needs to be done is to ensure that the perspective of the host community is incorporated into the evaluation process. Organizations dedicated to improving the health of poor communities around the world need to take into account community members' reports on what they see to be the benefits and costs in both the short and long term. They need to examine the actual outcomes and ask whether host communities are better off as a result of volunteer projects. And what types of programs produce the best outcomes? As Matt MacGregor says about Timmy Global Health's efforts to measure the impact of its programs, "Is this perfect? Of course not. But it's much better than simply referring a patient and hoping for the best."

Matt is correct: "hoping for the best" is never the ideal strategy when volunteer organizations spend their time and money in poor communities. Documenting the actual improvements in host communities, the presumed beneficiaries of the trips, is difficult but also essential for being able to claim that these activities are truly valuable.

10

Programmatic Focus

Principle 5: Focus on Prevention

The lack of investment in prevention is a challenge in the United States and elsewhere. Public health professionals as well as medical sociologists like me often cite the parable told by John McKinlay about the physician who compares himself to the person so busy saving people from drowning that he never has time to "refocus upstream" to figure out what is pushing them into the water in the first place.[1] The call to refocus upstream, to prevent illness by addressing its underlying causes, is a key theme in research and practice in public health. Yet in many health-related programs around the world, the attention is, understandably, on those already drowning.

Alexandra Martiniuk is an epidemiologist on medical school faculties in both Canada and Australia who has been researching health in poor countries. She and her colleagues analyzed volunteer efforts and point out that one of the key deficiencies in short-term medical missions is the lack of preventive services.[2]

Some volunteers are aware of this; medical volunteers working in the primary care clinics I participated in expressed this very concern. In Ecuador, almost all patients were suffering from aches, many due to work but some also to dehydration. The doctor emphasized with each patient the importance of drinking more water. Most patients weren't drinking much water. Some drank juice but not enough. This seemed related to their understanding that water can carry parasites.

A volunteer interpreter expressed frustration. "I always tell them the same story: all your pain will disappear if you drink more water. How could we make this more efficient? I don't know if there's a way, but it would help so many people if we could somehow spread this word of drinking more water without having to tell anybody else."

Spreading the word requires more than telling people what to do. It assumes the water is indeed safe to drink, an assurance impossible in much of the world. It is widely understood that addressing the need for clean water and effective sewage systems would prevent millions of deaths annually.[3] Yet the focus of the vast majority of investments in health, all over the world, is on trying to save the drowning, to treat people suffering from preventable illnesses.

One of the Ecuadorian partners commented on the need for a much broader range of public health and prevention measures. "Timmy has concentrated on curative treatments and not preventative. If they concentrate on preventative measures, it means tackling something deeper with educative talks, for example, in preventative measures against parasites, contraception and sex education, things for prevention on long-term issues."

Women's health issues were obvious candidates for a focus on prevention in clinics in Ecuador and Haiti, especially when women were thought by the clinicians to have sexually transmitted diseases or to have been victims of violence by their partners. The sponsoring organizations, though, seemed incapable of providing related services or advice; some staff mentioned local religious concerns about contraception.

Problems like these are universal and not easily alleviated.[4] Certainly, short-term volunteers are not going to solve them. But seeing the results of these problems without attention to prevention is frustrating for volunteers and certainly not best for patients. One Ecuadorean health professional suggested that the partnership of local and outside health providers could be doing a better job. "What about cases beyond that of physical and targeting the causes?" she asked. "For example, in a domestic abuse case we [Timmy and the hospital] can complement each other and provide for those needs. It's not only a mental problem but spiritual."

There are myriad underlying causes for illness in poor countries, from environmental degradation that makes malaria more prevalent[5] to malnutrition that increases the likelihood of death for children and pregnant women.[6] Organizations that devote great energy to curing disease one sick person at a time would accomplish even more by working with their partners to identify and then address underlying causes.

Principle 6: Integrate Diverse Types of Health Services

One common criticism of current health activities in the poorer countries is their fragmentation by disease—the "vertical" or "silo" approach that has a different program, staff, and funding mechanism for each health problem identified.[7] Short-term volunteering has the same problem: organizations tend to concentrate on one very specific surgical repair problem, or one type of cancer screening, or on primary health care limited to acute somatic symptoms, or on training in one particular area of interest—a phenomenon also referred to as the "organification" of medical care.[8] Global health advocates recommend a more comprehensive and integrated approach.[9] This is desirable in any context but especially where people must travel far, often by foot or expensive transport, for very sporadic and limited services.

Dental and eye care are high on the list of services that would, ideally, be integrated into primary care missions. There is a tremendous need for both, but they are rarely provided and not even usually included in the conversation.[10] Oral health is a serious problem in terms of pain, infection, and overall well-being but is unavailable in much of the world. Eye care, also rarely provided, is widely needed for vision correction, cataracts, and glaucoma. Even scarcer is mental health care, which is very difficult to provide in short-term encounters across cultural divides. Some international volunteer organizations do provide eyeglasses and cataract surgery or basic dental screening in sporadic outreach clinics,[11] and a very few do address mental health care, but they are mostly disconnected from other elements of health care.[12]

Valerie Matron, who works for Timmy Global Health in Quito, Ecuador, agrees on the goal of integrating health services and adds to the list of what's needed. "I think we should bring a physical therapist to all brigades, because everyone has so many physical ailments that I think even education on how they can do their jobs differently, how they can pick up things differently, I think all of those things will be extremely valuable. And then we need to solidify a partnership here for vision services and dentistry. That's what poor people want. They all want eyeglasses. You can't sew; you can't make your basket if you can't see the thread."

Granted, it is difficult enough to put together a surgical team with specialized surgeons, anesthesiologists, and operating room nurses or a primary care team with pharmacists, nurses, and physicians. The idea of integrating the equipment and staff required for ophthalmic and oral health screening and treatment into a primary care trip is surely daunting. But it is not impossible.

Dental, vision, and medical care are also entirely separated in countries that send volunteers, so it is not surprising that organizations rarely think about doing them together. Coordination among different specialties that do not normally work together would be difficult. But given the scarcity of resources in many host communities and the amount of time, money, and energy required by volunteer organizations and patients alike for each kind of mission, coordination is very much worth pursuing.

Principle 7: Build Local Capacity

Two-thirds of the organizations in my study indicated that their volunteers train local healthcare workers. "Capacity building" has become an important buzzword in the world of development, but what this actually means on the ground varies greatly. At the least, it should involve training staff members to help them develop professionally and personally so they can provide services even if the volunteer organization does not continue its activities or does not have programs year-round. Capacity building can also involve developing facilities such as laboratories and operating rooms, with the proviso they not be planted once with no follow-up and that equipment must continue to work and staffing and supplies be adequate.

Dr. Marc Levitt's program to train surgeons in pediatric colorectal surgery, described earlier, seems a very good example of the right kind of capacity building that can be done in some locations. His first volunteer experience was dissatisfying: he worried about the lack of an intensive care unit and proper medications for postsurgical care. In planning Colorectal Teams Overseas, he decided he would take surgical teams only to places with facilities for operating safely on children *and* where local surgeons could be trained to continue the work. "I would not do it without a host surgeon who is very engaged and capable," he told me. "Otherwise there is no point. We go with three surgical teams, operating in three ORs, and each OR has two people from our team and one local surgeon." Eva Levitt, CTO's patient relations coordinator, notes that videos of the operations are also streamed for other local health professionals to observe.

CTO takes a global view of building capacity, often including trainees from countries other than the host country. For example, when the CTO team went to Capetown, South Africa, twenty-four surgeons from around Africa joined them for the training, their flights paid for by Kind Cuts for Kids in Australia. Some surgeon trainees have also spent time in Cincinnati learning from Dr. Levitt's team at that city's children's hospital. Dr. Levitt stays in regular e-mail contact with the host surgeons and has also begun to evaluate the effects of the training on practice through pre- and posttesting.

The opposite of local capacity building happens far too often, especially when the volunteers' experience is considered the primary goal. For example, the representative of one sponsoring organization told me about student volunteers arriving in host countries, being given a quick orientation, and then "planning for a public health education session or delivering it." I wondered who guided the volunteers on how to develop a public health session. The answer was shocking. The field operations manager at the site, noting that volunteers "have access to the Internet," would simply assign volunteers to the task, asking, "Could you guys do some research and come up with a lesson plan for tomorrow for sex education for our adolescent group or something like that, or a healthy cooking habit?"

The idea of American students arriving in another country and almost immediately "teaching" local residents about sex or any other topic, based on Internet research, is appalling. Not only is it bad for the host community, but it isn't even good education for the volunteers, who may learn a very false lesson that they have some kind of special expertise—when in fact all they *really* have is access to the Web. They know very little about the lives of the people they are lecturing to, often including the language they speak.

One volunteer who had participated in this type of program told me about her frustration with the process. She wondered why the local interpreters and community health workers who know the community and the language were not being trained to deliver the educational sessions to community members themselves. Instead, they were relegated to the role of interpreters for newly arrived and naive outsiders.

Partner staff members must play an essential role. "I've learned over the years," said one NGO director. "I don't allow Americans to give the prescriptions to the patient. I have a trained pharmacist who does that teaching, so they work with the Americans who are filling the prescriptions, but she's the one, she's providing education to that patient at the same time, not just saying one tab, three times a day in broken Spanish or Creole."

Valerie Matron offered a similar example.

> Vicky and Marielena [staff members of partner Tierra Nueva Foundation] are assigned to different communities," she explains, "Timmy visits ten communities, and Vicky is responsible for five for the follow-up, and Marielena is responsible for the other five. They know a lot more of the patients. So when we go on brigades, Vicky always goes to the same ones and Marielena always goes to the same ones. At pharmacy time, when you get your medication, Vicky and Marielena are sitting there. They're the ones giving out the medication and they know you. You come, and you're a hypertensive, and they check your blood pressure, and if it's doing well they congratulate you. If it's not doing so well, they talk to you like you're family.

Hiring and (when needed) training members of host communities to carry out many of the important activities of a volunteer organization have much value. Yet financial constraints or the desire to involve more volunteers may limit this, to the detriment of the program and the morale of host community members. For example, in the Amazon Basin villages in Ecuador, local staff members sometimes felt left out, despite important jobs they might have assumed. For example, the interpreters were almost all Americans, although they had no training in medical language or interpreting and in some cases had just arrived in the country. Their job was to interpret for patients and physicians, from English into Spanish and back again, but if the patient did not speak Spanish, a local interpreter would then translate from the American's Spanish to Kichwa, the local indigenous language, and then do the reverse when the patient spoke.

This approach saves money by not having to pay local interpreters, but it risks compromising quality of care. One of the Ecuadorean community health workers offered an alternative that would require a longer-range investment. "I would like to have the volunteers come and give us courses in English in order to communicate with the doctors and those who care for people here in Ecuador."

I heard about and observed many instances in which volunteers were doing work that could be much better performed by community members who spoke the language, knew the situation, and were not there for only a week or two. For example, community members in Uganda who translated the community health lessons delivered by newly arrived volunteers would have been much more effective in the role of teachers themselves. Involving local staff members in identifying needs and solutions and in providing core services can improve quality. At the same time it offers an educational model for volunteers that does not privilege their (often limited) knowledge and skills over those of their hosts.

Principle 8: Strengthen Volunteer Preparation

In looking at the "career" of a volunteer, from initial interest through application, selection, preparation, and adaptation, we see that the typical volunteer-sponsoring organization recruits on the Internet or through its own educational or church institution and accepts most people who apply. Many, if not most, programs provide grossly insufficient preparation for volunteers when it comes to the history, culture, and language of the country they will be visiting, as well as the work they will be doing. Most organizations send volunteers with limited preparation into unfamiliar environments; volunteers are provided basic information about the country and travel requirements and then put into work situations almost immediately upon arrival.

This may work reasonably well after the first couple of days if the sending and the host organizations have procedures to orient, incorporate, and supervise these largely ill-prepared volunteers in the work they will be doing. But local partners for volunteer programs do not always exist. Good procedures for incorporating newcomers into new environments and work situations are not always in place. And after the first couple of days, many volunteers are already halfway through their stay. Some host country staff and some volunteers confirmed that they see this as a real problem that needs to be addressed.

Of course, it is unlikely that a short-term volunteer will be able to learn a new language or gain a thorough understanding of a new country before traveling. Still, it is important that sending organizations emphasize being able to use some basic terms of greeting, knowing something about the country, and perhaps most important, learning how to act with a sense of cultural humility when meeting people whose lives are very different from those of the volunteers.

For organizations whose goal is to transform volunteer lives by creating an opportunity for intercultural understanding and future global health leadership, the preparation and follow-up must both be extensive and thoughtful. Amizade's approach, described in chapter 3, is unusual, but approaches that involve in-depth study and reflection about history, culture, and international development have been shown to enhance significantly the long-term benefit of a trip for the volunteers.[13] Such preparation, though, is less likely to be feasible for specialized surgical missions and may be more suited to students or other volunteers who can participate in a more in-depth program of preparation and follow-up.

Another aspect of volunteer preparation that is typically ignored is the opportunity to impart what previous volunteers have learned from their experiences. Having each new group work with the previous one to learn the ropes could significantly reduce the time new volunteers must spend adapting to the country and work environment, potentially allowing them to spend that time more productively, be more effective, and make fewer errors. I found few instances in which programs organize a clear transmission of knowledge gained by the previous group as each new group adapts and figures out ways of doing its work, whether in clinic or in laboratory training—but experience in any number of situations suggests that such programs would go a long way toward strengthening volunteer participation.

Though it would be logistically challenging, having an overlapping time between groups would allow departing volunteers to share with new arrivals what they have learned from their very recent experience. Many organizations have full-time local staffers who orient new volunteers, which is critical, but they cannot personally guide every member of a new group and after a while may take many of the day-to-day routines for granted.

The possibility that something—indeed, many things—might go wrong during the trip and that the benefits might be limited certainly exists under circumstances in which inexperienced, untrained, or unprepared people arrive in a new country on a weekend afternoon, meet a host family or have a day for tourism, and then launch into activity on Monday morning for five days (or perhaps a couple of weeks), returning home the following weekend. Thus the length of trips is an important consideration, as are the selection and preparation of volunteers.

Principle 9: Have Volunteers Stay Longer

Host-country staffs and longer-term expatriate staffs regard short-term stays of less than three weeks (in some views, less than six months or a year) as not being especially valuable. Short-term volunteers, in addition to often being ill prepared and inexperienced, require time to learn how to function well and relate better to the host communities so that the volunteering experience is mutually beneficial. Some make an exception for the brief but well-organized intensive surgical visits in emergency situations or in situations that allow for follow-up, but the perspective that volunteer trips should be longer in order to be beneficial is pretty universal.

Even fans of the short-term surgical trip would ideally want it to be more regular or at least be sure it makes significant additional contributions. For example, a surgeon in Ghana who worked with the pediatric colorectal team from Cincinnati told interviewer Caroline Kusi that the value of the CTO approach was that the volunteers were able to operate for much longer hours and treat more children, which cut down the waiting list for patients. With other surgical visitors, the results are less satisfying: "When a volunteer comes and does jobs on a day-to-day basis without an increase of operating time or anything of that sort, that will not make much of a difference." Even with the CTO team, he expressed the wish that they would not just arrive for one week and then be gone. "To make a significant difference, [volunteerism] will have to be long-term," said the surgeon. "We offload our colorectal cases; yes, that is good, it is beneficial to the patients, beneficial to the nation as a whole, and beneficial to us. That is good, but if we had it more frequently, then that would reduce the waiting list significantly."

While some organizations are considering cutting back or eliminating short-term volunteering (discussed in the next chapter) as they recognize the limited value of short trips, there are still compelling reasons from the sending organizations' perspective to continue to sponsor trips of one or two weeks, making the shift to longer stays a difficult principle. For instance, many professionals, especially in the United States, have very limited vacation time and cannot be away from work or family for longer periods. And shorter visits mean that more people can be included in volunteer trips. This is advantageous for the organizations because it allows them to involve more people in their activities and thus provide the benefits envisioned for volunteers, who also potentially become supporters of the organization upon their return.

On top of this, there are more direct financial considerations. As a rule, three-week trips do not generate three times as much revenue for an organization as one-week trips. For those organizations that rely on fees to support their operations or generate profits, more volunteers for shorter trips means more income. Unite for Sight provides a good illustration: the group widely advertises for one-week volunteers to assist with its outreach clinics in Ghana, accepts almost everyone who can pay the $1,500 program fee plus all their expenses, and then uses this money to pay for its programming.

Nevertheless, consistent with the findings of Benjamin Lough in his interviews in Kenya,[14] host staff members in my research are quite clear about the inferior value of very short-term volunteers. I agree. I think a better case can be made for a one-week mission of surgical or other specialty teams, if properly organized and with follow-up care assured, than for one-week trips by untrained students and church members, which require a higher proportion of time for adapting and provide only limited or questionable benefits to volunteers and hosts alike.

CONCLUSION

Lessons Learned; Responding to the Debate

> There is something highly problematic about service that "uses" encounters
> with tragedy and poverty as a means to any ends other than the alleviation of
> suffering, either directly or indirectly.
>
> —JASON KIMELMAN-BLOCH

One day during my last stage of finishing this book, my e-mail inbox
began to fill up as friends and colleagues forwarded to me an opinion piece
posted to Aljazeera.com. It was the latest critique of international volunteering, another discussion of the "white-savior industrial complex."[1]

These sorts of articles appear more frequently than ever as the number
of volunteer trips continues to grow. While many people consider volunteering altruistic, as something that accomplishes good, the criticisms are
wide-ranging: cultural insensitivity, self-serving motivations, perpetuation
of inequalities, and lack of preparation, follow-up, and understanding of
what is most needed. Critics point to myriad possible ill effects—medical,
political, economic, cultural—on host communities.

What are we to make of all this criticism? It seems unfair to be so hard
on people acting on their passion or faith to benefit others, who spend their
time and money on the cause of better health in underserved communities.
After all, there is an abundance of anecdotal and other evidence that these
volunteer visits improve lives (some of it reported in chapter 6). Would it
be better if the tens of thousands of people who have begun NGOs to work
in specific communities or to combat specific diseases simply stayed home

or spent their overseas travel time exclusively as tourists? Would it be better if the hundreds of thousands of students, dentists, teachers, surgeons, nurses, and ministers never spent time in clinics or hospitals in poor countries, where the needs are so great?

These questions pose precisely the dilemma faced in examining short-term volunteering. Without careful evaluation and follow-up, it is difficult to know whether it is better or worse for poor communities to receive short-term volunteers from other countries. And what are the alternatives?

A more nuanced assessment is needed that promotes the best volunteering practices and identifies those lacking value. The purpose of this book has been to contribute to that understanding. My conclusions are consistent with the advice offered by Dr. Ian Smith, who along with his family worked in Nepal for sixteen years as a medical missionary:

> I think there are ways of making short-term volunteerism more effective by putting it into the context of long-term, locally planned, locally owned support. I think the risk is when you keep it totally external and parachute people in to work for a few weeks and give them the sense that they've made a major contribution. In fact sometimes it can even be damaging, particularly if it distorts local economies, if it's disempowering, if it's raising expectations, it's creating precedence that is then very difficult to sustain, all those sorts of damaging aspects.

Today Smith advises the director-general of the World Health Organization, although the views above are his own and not the WHO's position. As he asserts, there *are* ways to make short-term volunteering more valuable to host communities and allay some of the criticisms. My own findings and other research support his view.

In previous chapters, I explored in detail specific problems with current practices and potential ways to alleviate some of the concerns. I think it's valuable to reconsider here some important points in the overall debate.

Opportunity Costs

Volunteers and the organizations that sponsor them spend billions of dollars each year in time, equipment, transportation, and administrative costs. We must ask not only whether it is money well spent but also whether it could be spent more directly and productively to support existing programs and personnel within the poorer countries. For example, Becton Dickinson spent an estimated $2 million to send employees to Ghana as volunteers on three occasions for three weeks each time.[2] Another group of forty volunteers each spent nearly $2,000, supplemented by considerable fund-raising, to work for five days in clinics in Ecuador. Those large sums benefit American staff and U.S airlines and to a considerably less extent the host economies, and they are only two examples among thousands of programs. It is very tempting to ask what else might have been accomplished had the money been sent directly to the host partner.

Of course, the reality is that without the opportunity to travel and encounter new places, without the possibility of a hands-on experience of helping, and, for some, without the gratification of receiving others' admiration, volunteers and donors would simply not spend their funds in this way. "Just send the money" is an unrealistic alternative. For many sponsor organizations, the volunteer experience is a large part of the value of their programs. Still, the question must be asked. And from all we have seen, the answer has to be that the money is not being spent in the wisest and most productive way possible.

The Ethics of Medical Volunteering

The ethical issues in medical volunteering, discussed in chapter 7, are worth revisiting. Probably the most widely published criticisms of short-term health volunteering come from medical journals, with authors questioning the ethics of having medical or premedical students do things they would clearly not be permitted to practice in their own countries—and where the benefits to hosts are anything but obvious.[3] This problem is at least as great when volunteers have no health background whatsoever.

Dr. Lani K. Ackerman, writing about the ethics of short-term health electives in developing countries, notes, "While there is little doubt that these electives have student support, and represent times of personal and professional enthusiasm about medicine, there is little literature evaluating the educational effects, much less the ethical issues inherent in these experiences."[4] She raises a range of ethical issues: potential harm to the host population; health and safety risks for students during their travel, such as from infectious disease, traffic accidents, and crime; and guilt over bad outcomes from unsupervised and unskilled practice of medicine.

In response to these concerns, the Working Group on Ethics Guidelines for Global Health Training (WEIGHT) was established at Duke University, and guidelines it developed are now part of pretrip orientation for health professional students at several schools.[5] Some institutions, though, have not yet gotten on board. In fact, many of the very sending institutions for which the guidelines are intended assume they do not apply to them and therefore make no effort to follow them.[6]

When undergraduate students with no medical training and medical students with minimal clinical experience act as physicians—diagnosing patients and providing them with medication—the ethical problems should be obvious. Yet even experienced physicians come in for criticism. A group of surgeons from the Uniformed Services University of the Health Sciences expounded on "the seven sins of humanitarian medicine":[7]

Sin No. 1: Leaving a mess behind
Sin No. 2: Failing to match technology to local needs and abilities
Sin No. 3: Failing of NGOs to cooperate and help each other
Sin No. 4: Failing to have a follow-up plan
Sin No. 5: Allowing politics, training, or other distracting goals to trump
   service, while representing the mission as "service"
Sin No. 6: Going where we are not wanted or needed and/or being poor
   guests
Sin No. 7: Doing the right thing for the wrong reason

Surgical interventions with inadequate follow-up (sin no. 4) can leave patients behind with no one to treat postsurgical complications, thus causing actual harm. Some medical missions have even brought (or groups have sent) nonfunctioning equipment or expired medications.[8]

Many of these problems are likely unintentional, but they are also not surprising in the all-too-common situations in which local communities are not seriously involved in planning and no evaluation is carried out to consider both pluses and negatives of medical missions.

Religion's Role

Another critique of international volunteering is its strong religious missionary element. The role of religion is complicated. As Linda Polman observes, "The world of do-it-yourself aid is deeply haunted by the spirit
of the priests of yore. Religious MONGOs, especially those based in the
United States, are the fastest-growing branch of the aid industry."[9] As we
saw earlier, the place of faith in medical trips can be very subtle or quite
overt, going so far as to include preaching and praying as part of a clinic or
showing patients films about the life of Jesus.[10]

Nancy Gard McGehee and Kathleen Andereck looked at volunteer
tourism in Tijuana, Mexico, and concluded, "The role of organized religion in volunteer tourism often seems to be the 'elephant in the living
room' that no one wishes to discuss."[11] They criticize evangelical tourism
for deliberately trying to change local culture; they found Tijuana residents are least likely to prefer volunteers from faith-based organizations.

Faith-based missions, though, must be recognized for providing a great
deal of medical care in remote and underserved areas. Religious motivation
inspires many people to give their time, even their lives, to humanitarian
causes. In some cases, the host-community members are devout Christians
themselves and welcome outsiders who share their faith. Additionally, liberation theology, with its emphasis on social justice, offers a very important
model for addressing the underlying causes of ill health in solidarity with
poor communities.[12] Some religious thinkers and leaders have challenged
the inequities and power abuses that contribute to so much disease and
misery in the world. However, in those cases when conversion is the primary goal and health care the means for achieving it, faith-based volunteer
missions become objectionable, in my view. Healing bodies as a pretext
for saving souls, rather than as the primary mission in the case of most
faith-based organizations, is deceptive and potentially coercive.

A New Colonialism?

In the introduction, I referred to authors who consider volunteering to be
a new form of colonialism. Earlier forms of colonialism involved extracting raw materials, often by force, from conquered territories to fuel the

Industrial Revolution, advance the development of the colonizing nations, and increase the wealth and comfort of the colonial masters. Today's volunteers might use their experiences in poor countries to build careers, social capital, and personal satisfaction. It is possible to see some similarities between these two types of "extractions" of benefits from poor countries.

Early colonizers prided themselves on bringing the benefits of "civilization" to "heathen" lands. As do volunteers today, they claimed they did good work. Indeed, colonial doctors were thanked and appreciated by people whose lives they saved. But colonial rulers used medical care to appease and win over the native peoples who resisted their rule. As an early French document asserted, "For the conquering and pacifying army . . . the doctor is the most necessary and precious collaborator. . . . Our colonial leaders . . . have willingly replaced regiments or battalions of occupation with a dispensary or a hospital."[13]

Today the Peace Corps is explicit that one of its two primary goals is to promote positive feelings about Americans; the Brookings Institution promotes volunteers as "the best diplomats" from the United States.[14] The relationship is hardly as coercive as colonialism, but to some extent today's volunteers are still (and usually unwittingly) serving the political agendas of their governments in addition to providing services.

To be sure, there are dissenting voices. Jim Butcher and Peter Smith, two researchers from England, dismiss the comparison: "It is wrong to argue that today's tourist fantasies mimic those of colonial times or that volunteer tourism presumes westernization as a part of the development process. It is hard to agree that today's volunteers believe they are there to 'bring civilization to the natives.'"[15]

Of course, the language has changed—today's volunteers do not talk about "civilizing the natives." But some speak of their missions as "saving the unchurched." And even for those not preaching salvation, the phenomenon, as I see it, still has many of the same qualities. People with formal education and many financial advantages want to bring Western practices to the poor and uneducated and show them how to do things the "right" way. Add to this that the volunteers and their sponsor organizations and home countries all gain many benefits from these activities.

So it is not completely far-fetched to compare the extraction of advantages from the poor by today's well-off brigade members (yes, including researchers such as myself) to the past and current activities of Western

powers in extracting raw materials and human labor from the same countries to serve their own purposes. They also reinforce their own relative advantage back home by gaining career-related experience and connections.

Yet—and it is a big yet—it is exceedingly difficult, perhaps even wrong-
headed, to argue that alleviating pain, preventing disease, and surgically
correcting life-threatening problems should be construed as nefarious.
This is one of the central dilemmas and important challenges for those
who earnestly seek to reduce health disparities and alleviate suffering
around the world. They must consider how this can be done in the most
effective way possible, without reinforcing the vast inequalities between
and within nations and while keeping the interests of poor communities
always as the top priority.

Do Motives Matter?

I was not very surprised to discover that international health volunteers
often have many motivations other than contributing to the health of people in poor communities: adventure, international exposure, bragging
rights, personal fulfillment, résumé building, exotic travel, and others.
I was, perhaps naively, more surprised by how frequently the organizations that sponsor these missions also have other motivations. I had a pretty
good idea that short-term trips, on their own, do not accomplish as much
for the host communities' health as organizers hope or claim. I wasn't as
prepared for the reality that too often health benefits for host communities
are *intentionally* only part of the picture. Enhancing their own reputations;
offering educational and service experiences to students, employees, and
church members; bringing Jesus to non-Christians; making money—these
are all part of the picture.

Organizers often told me their goal was partly or entirely to provide
travelers with a valuable educational experience or opportunity to serve
others, which they believed would occur automatically simply by virtue of
their participation. In many cases, they were quite explicit in their expecta-
tion (or hope) that volunteers would return with greater cultural awareness and skills and make important contributions at home as advocates for
social justice.[16]

It should be no surprise, then, that organizations generally do an in-adequate job of preparing volunteers and a much worse job of evaluating project outcomes. Not only are thorough preparation and systematic eval-uation difficult and therefore subsumed under the more pressing concerns related to trip logistics, but they are rarely considered very important. Even organizations whose focus is entirely on providing the best possible benefit to their hosts do little to document their successes. Value is assumed.

Volunteers' experiences tend to have a high value for organizations and scholars alike. For example, Matt Baillie Smith and Nina Laurie, two pro-fessors in England who study international development, argue that "in-ternational volunteering may promote global equity by fostering greater awareness of social justice and development and enhancing global citizen-ship, or promote corporate efficiency and career progression through in-dividual skills enhancement."[17] They don't say how, nor do they articulate the benefits to host communities.

Jim Butcher and Peter Smith also focus on the volunteers in their study of voluntourism. "It can be argued," they write, "that the contribution to development cannot be measured simply in terms of the projects them-selves. Rather, the projects play a role in developing people who will, in the course of their careers and lives, act ethically in favour of those less well-off."[18]

Despite all this hope that volunteers will be transformed in a way that will benefit the world, we have seen that even this outcome must be ques-tioned. The evidence for it is still quite limited. Yes, there is value in the opportunity for people with privilege to gain greater cultural understand-ing and commitment to social justice, but they must also understand the potential costs associated with short service trips to other countries. Some volunteers find themselves transformed by their experiences and devote themselves to lifelong service, but the majority apparently return home with, at best, fond memories of voluntourism and, at worst, reinforced prejudices and false impressions. Still, even if we could *prove* that volun-teers do become more aware and responsible global citizens and advocates for social justice on behalf of the poor, this outcome cannot justify the po-tential cost to host communities of poorly designed volunteer trips.

So, do individual or organizational motives matter? This question takes us back to the basic concerns about the validity of international health volunteering. What if a volunteer does go on a trip mostly to have a great story to tell, or is motivated by the "white-savior industrial complex"? What if an organization sponsors trips primarily because they look good to prospective employees or students or promote an evangelical mission? What if the *doing* of service is what counts the most, rather than, or as much as, improvements in the health and well-being of poor communities? Does this mean that they cannot also provide valuable, even lifesaving, health care services in poor communities?

Of course they can and often do provide valuable services. But I strongly believe that to treat the volunteer's experience or the organization's reputation or religious priorities as on a par with, or even more important than, the benefits to hosts is to exploit poor communities for the benefit of people from wealthier countries. And these other goals, as we saw earlier, can conflict with or reduce the focus on achieving the most effective results for host communities.

Rabbi Jason Kimelman-Block offered a strong view on this issue in a 2010 opinion piece. He wrote, "There is something highly problematic about service that 'uses' encounters with tragedy and poverty as a means to any ends other than the alleviation of suffering, either directly or indirectly."[19] This opinion seems quite categorical until you consider whether "indirectly" might refer to the possibility of influencing young people to become advocates and leaders for the alleviation of suffering in the long term, as some organizations claim as their goal. So I contacted him and he agreed to the possibility of this benefit, but added that the organization must be very purposeful in teaching the volunteers about advocacy, not just assume it will happen automatically.

I'm OK with it being multiple steps away. This person may be a sustained activist and will continue to be in solidarity with marginalized communities. But it's on the trip organizers and leaders to show how they are connecting the dots for people, making sure it happens, not expect that it will somehow just happen.

I think that service trips have value when they are done from a solidarity perspective, and that is less common. If service is a means to an end and not about the people in the community they are working with, if it is just about *my* experience, what it does for *me*, there is an objectification going on. I worry about objectification.

These observations contribute to the case for longer trips as part of continuous programs. Longer-term programs with fewer participants can be more selective and can take the time to train volunteers and orient them to the work and the environment. This approach benefits not only the volunteers but also the host communities. When volunteers are skilled and prepared for their missions, when the tasks they undertake are well suited to those skills, and when they are working in an environment with well-established procedures and effective supervision, the chances are greater that they will accomplish something of value to hosts.

The evidence from previous studies suggests that longer exposure to international experiences has a longer-lasting effect on volunteers. This should come as no surprise. Further, embedding the volunteering experience in an educational program that prepares volunteers beforehand and builds on the experience afterward is most likely to produce such effects.[20] Very few organizations do either: the great majority of volunteer experiences are brief, with minimal preparation and follow-up.

Matt MacGregor agrees with the importance of purposeful preparation.

The *big myth* [my emphasis] in this work is that everyone who goes on an international trip is immediately changed, they have a transformed life and when they come back, they become a health advocate. The truth is it that this is definitely possible, but it is much more possible if it's done within a larger structure where you help someone who has traveled abroad maintain a focus on those issues when you come back to your campus. Without that, many volunteers state that they've had this transformational experience at the end of the trip but there is no tangible change in their attitudes, beliefs, or actions that demonstrate that.

Perhaps these are issues primarily for students. Perhaps it doesn't matter whether a surgeon or dentist who spends a week doing thirty hernia operations or colorectal repairs or tooth extractions returns home with greater cultural sensitivity or international awareness. These programs tend to be very focused on the tasks and much less on the value to the specialists. It may well be that a focus on changing the volunteers is more salient when what they have to offer is very limited.

The insistence on giving primary consideration to the needs of host communities is evident in the writings of Partners in Health cofounder

Paul Farmer, who embraces the Preferential Option for the Poor (POP)—a concept developed in the context of Catholic liberation theology.[21] The needs of the poor should take precedence over any other priorities.

The bioethicists Solomon Benatar, Abdallah Daar, and Peter Singer disagree with the arguments made by Farmer and others. "In arguing that it is both desirable and necessary to develop a global mindset in health ethics," they write, "we suggest that this change need not be based merely on altruism, and that promoting long-term self-interest is also essential if we acknowledge that lives across the world are inextricably interlinked by forces that powerfully shape health and wellbeing."[22]

The research shows overwhelmingly that altruism is rarely the sole motivation in volunteering, regardless of the activity or context. Granted, it may be impossible to expect people to have only one motive for any specific behavior, and it is very likely not necessary for the accomplishment of effective work to have no other goals than the work itself. The complexity of human life is such that some people who embark on an activity for entirely self-serving reasons may indeed have their lives changed. People join causes all the time as a result of circumstances and social ties, only to have that initial contact evolve later into advocacy—even around issues as highly charged as abortion.[23] The young man I quoted in chapter 4 who went on a health brigade only to follow an attractive woman later became a full-time staff person working in another country to promote health.

Acknowledging the realities and complexities of human behavior does not mean, however, that we should not be concerned about the potential conflict in goals at the organizational level. Matt MacGregor struggled with this tension in our conversation. He offers a valuable perspective.

> How do we balance the value to the volunteer with the value to the person on the ground? The trick of organizations that do this well should be getting them both to benefit as mutually as possible and that means thinking clearly through what structures need to be in place to support these communities and these patients. It's not enough to say, "Oh, but my point is to transform the lives of volunteers." If you're doing that at the expense of someone else, it's not a wonderful thing to do. If you're doing that in a way that benefits mutually, then that's a powerful thing.

This emphasis on mutuality brings us back to the first principle of effective trips described earlier. If a volunteer trip is designed to build solidarity and contribute to a more just world, as Kimelman-Block advocates, it can indeed be powerful. Every trip organizer and prospective volunteer needs to consider how to achieve these goals while always staying focused on the POP. Surely meeting the needs of poor and oppressed people must be the foremost objective for all involved in volunteer projects.

Discontinue Short-Term Trips?

One way to improve the effectiveness of volunteer health activities would be to incorporate the critical components of good volunteer trips, the nine principles prescribed in earlier chapters. Yet very few organizations follow most of the principles. If an organization cannot follow at least several of these basic requirements, if it cannot show that its programs provide as much value for the host communities as might justify the enormous investment of financial and human resources, it should seriously consider abandoning the idea of short-term volunteer trips altogether. Alternatively, it could be made clearer to poor communities that since the mission is not primarily about improving their lives, they will be compensated appropriately for what they are contributing to the visiting organizations and volunteers.

Some organizations have indeed chosen to reduce or eliminate short-term volunteer programs. As Dr. Ian Smith told me, "We've not seen this as being the primary strategy for resolving the issues." Indeed, the WHO does not use short-term volunteers. "We tend to look primarily at the needs of countries in terms of what can be done to help them build their national capacities," explains Dr. Smith, "so we're very much working with ministries of health, ministries of education, etc. to help build up their national capacity rather than seeing the solution as being meeting gaps by sending out large numbers of volunteers from developed countries."

Other organizations have reconsidered the short-term trip and limit their activities to longer-term missions or to sending paid professionals. That is the approach taken by Partners in Health, a highly respected organization based at Harvard University with health projects in many parts of the world. PIH has only a few positions for *specialized* volunteers and expects them to commit for a period of at least several months.

"We generally do not recruit volunteers for overseas work," PIH explains on its website. "Local medical professionals and community health workers at our partner projects carry out the bulk of the work, and language barriers and our limited resources for supervision and training also prevent us from accommodating volunteers. While on occasion we do engage volunteer medical and technical specialists, we're committed to working with the members of the communities we serve in order to expand local skills and knowledge, build up local infrastructure, and ensure sustainability."[24]

Two of the best-known international medical programs—Médecins sans Frontières (MSF, or Doctors Without Borders in English) and the International Committee of the Red Cross (ICRC)—rely on paid professionals willing to spend a minimum of several months, rather than taking volunteers. It is interesting to note that when I talk about my research informally, people almost invariably ask whether I am referring to Doctors without Borders, since it is very well known for international medical work.[25] But MSF has adopted a very different model from the one I have been examining. Both MSF and ICRC respond to what are called "complex humanitarian emergencies" that result from armed conflicts as well as to natural disasters—situations that are not conducive to receiving short-term volunteers except for highly specialized people. MSF pays a monthly salary to the doctors, nurses, and other healthcare professionals who work on its missions and provides transportation, housing, pensions, and other benefits as well.

Some MSF staff members make brief visits after an emergency to organize the initial response work, according to Dr. Annick Antierens, MSF-Switzerland's deputy medical director, and some professionals spend only a few months filling in personnel gaps. But most MSF trips are much longer. "The big majority are still people who stay for six months or more," she says. "They cannot go if they don't stay for six months. The exceptions that would go for a very short time are extremely highly specialized people who would go for support or implementation [such as] anesthesiologists, surgeons, and gynecologists. These people, they are willing to help and do a mission but they cannot go for six months. Even these exceptional specialists are expected to stay at least four to six weeks."

Paying everyone is also the policy of the ICRC, whose "staff are remunerated professionals, and the ICRC does not have unpaid volunteers," says

Dr. Paul Bouvier, a senior medical adviser based in Geneva. "We work in situations of war and armed conflicts, in assistance and protection, including detention activities, in situations of violence which require strong expertise, experience and professionalism. For the ICRC, it was not possible and acceptable to send anyone without strong experience, high skills, and training into situations with major needs and high security risks."

Even some faith-based organizations that have over the years sponsored thousands of short-term volunteers are now reconsidering their practices. In the wake of its 2012 strategic planning process, the American Jewish World Service decided to limit the number of alternative spring break trips and focus on longer-term placements of volunteers in fewer countries. "We were concerned about the impact of the one-week program," Aaron Acharya of AJWS told me. "A lot of money spent. Great for volunteers but [questionable value] afterward."

People involved in short-term Christian missionary service trips have also questioned their value.[26] For example, Robert Reese, who was a missionary in Zimbabwe for two decades, concluded in his dissertation research that the "avalanche" of short-term volunteers traveling to poor countries serves to reinforce dependency in those countries. He is just one of those involved in medical mission work rethinking the best way to support real improvements in poor countries.[27] Many people who responded to the Catholic Health Association study expressed this same concern about dependency; indeed, one in four was not sure that short-term "medical missions" are very valuable for host communities.[28] Corbett and Fikkert address medical missionaries specifically when they caution about "when helping hurts" and offer suggestions on avoiding harm to both poor people and volunteers.[29]

Should short-term trips be discontinued? People who have thought carefully about this are questioning their value, and, as we have seen, some organizations are curtailing them in favor of a different model of volunteering that lasts longer and incorporates some of the key principles of effective volunteering outlined in the previous chapters. I concur with that preference as a much more cost-effective approach with a greater likelihood of positive impact.

Nevertheless, I believe that some short trips can be valuable (even if not as efficient or effective as longer trips) if they are carefully planned and focused, bring scarce and much-needed skills to a community, and involve evaluation and follow-up. They can have value especially if they are embedded in an ongoing service framework that provides continuity of care.

While the benefits to host communities remain to be documented more systematically, it would be wrong and unfair to discount completely the many examples of volunteers' contributions—the thousands of individuals regaining sight or being able to work or go to school or avoiding future cancers or having pain alleviated or feeling cared about. These examples are inspiring, and they surely motivate organizations and volunteers to continue their work.

In many cases, the health benefits contributed by short-term volunteers clearly improve and even save lives. The emphasis needs to be on maximizing these effects in the most responsible manner possible. For the most part, that means longer trips, much better volunteer preparation, and programs that are coordinated with and support local communities and officials on an ongoing basis, focus on underlying causes of ill health, and are embedded in continuous community-based assessment, partnership, and follow-up evaluation. In pursuit of a more just world, can we accept anything less?

Appendix A

Methods of Study

The research that formed the basis for this book included a survey of 177 United States-based organizations that sponsor short-term international volunteer trips that include health programs; 119 interviews with sponsors, host-country staff members, global health experts, and expatriates who have worked with volunteers in poor countries; and participant observation on two short-term trips and at orientation meetings before and evaluation meetings following five different trips. Detailed descriptions of each method follows.

Organizational Survey

The population of interest for our study was organizations that send volunteers abroad to do health-related work on a short-term basis, and our goal was to survey the entire population as far as feasible rather than to create a sample of such organizations. In order to be included, the organization had to meet four criteria: (1) it had to be based in the United States or staffed by Americans; (2) it placed volunteers or students outside the United States; (3) its service had a health component; (4) placement opportunities were available for six months or less.

There may be thousands of organizations that meet these criteria, and to our knowledge there is no comprehensive list. Many volunteer trips are created by individual churches or university faculty members and thus would be difficult to include. In order to identify as many organizations as possible that met our criteria, we carried out an extensive Internet-based search. We used Google as a search engine and employed a variety of search terms: "international health volunteering," "Christian health volunteering," "religious health volunteering," "global health volunteering," "corporate global health volunteering," "international health fellowships," "international health educational opportunities," "global health director, "international service learning," "global health elective," "medical school international internships," "intercultural nursing," "global health volunteer projects university," and "international volunteer organizations."

We explored the search engine results for links indicative of organizations that met our criteria. We determined (often through their mission statements and "About Us" sections) whether or not the organization or program fit the inclusion criteria. The websites discovered often led us to other international service volunteering programs and educational institutions; we used this information to investigate more groups, programs, and institutions to add to our list.

Some websites provided links to existing lists of international volunteer opportunities abroad, and we used these as guides to research more organizations. Useful sources included the University of Arizona (http://www.globalhealth.arizona.edu), International Health Volunteers (http://www.internationalhealthvolunteers.org), North Carolina State University Health Professions Advising Center (http://harvest.cals.ncsu.edu/health_pac/index.cfm?pageID=854) and Medical Mission Finder (http://www.missionfinder.org/medical). Medical Mission Exchange (www.mmex.org) has a database of short- and long-term medical missions serving the Dominican Republic, Guatemala, Haiti, Honduras, and Belize.

Word-of-mouth was an additional source for discovering new organizations throughout our research period; it is noteworthy that many people we know or met (mostly people not involved in health volunteering) mentioned organizations that they had heard about (my friend went with . . .) that did not appear in our Internet search. The constant discovery of new organizations led both to an expansion of the list and also to a strong awareness of its limits.

Once we identified an organization by any of these methods, we added it to our list and searched the website for specific information pertaining to our research question. We separated organizations into five categories: faith-based NGOs, educational and medical institutions, NGOs (not faith-based), corporate organizations, and brokers and voluntourism agencies.

The next step was to obtain an e-mail address for each organization in order to contact it to request participation in the survey. In many cases, there was no e-mail address listed, but the organization provided a contact form to be filled out by people interested in learning more about volunteer opportunities. We completed all such forms and used the e-mail address that responded to this form as our contact. If there was no response to the contact form within several days, we called the organization's office and asked for an e-mail contact. We called each organization twice and left messages if no one answered. These efforts yielded additional contact information.

During May to August of 2012, we sent e-mails to all 702 organizations on our list for which we were able to obtain e-mail contact information, asking people to connect to our survey on SurveyMonkey.com. Twenty-six wrote back saying they do not support short-term volunteers; these were removed from the initial list. If an organization's e-mail bounced back, and if upon further Internet investigation or unsuccessful use of alternative e-mails, we determined that it no longer existed, we removed it from the list; sixty-five more organizations were eliminated as a result. We sent two follow-up e-mail reminders to all 611 remaining organizations for which we had no indication (either from e-mail response or because they voluntarily listed their names in the survey form) whether or not they had replied.

The 611 organizations, the total number that we presumed to be valid (i.e., we did not receive a message saying the e-mail could not be delivered), included 316 faith-based NGOs, 70 educational institutions, 195 non-faith-based NGOs, and 30 voluntourism agencies.

Of these, four people responded by e-mail indicating that they were not willing to fill out the survey. Two hundred twenty-two (36.3%) did follow the link to the survey, but three of those checked "no" in response to the consent form and therefore were not able to continue. Of the 219 who agreed to the consent terms, there were quite a few who did not proceed with the survey. Two hundred five answered the first question, and 160 went through to the end as recorded by Survey Monkey (although these did not all respond to all the questions). We include in this analysis the 177 respondents who completed the survey at least as far as the sections describing the organization type, number of volunteers, countries included, and activities of volunteers. Thus the following results are based on those 177 respondents, who comprise 29 percent of the 611 we presume (but cannot be sure) received the request to participate.

Only four respondents identified themselves as being volunteer matching services; on the basis of other information they provided, we reclassified them with one of the other categories. The final sample thus comprised 89 faith-based organizations, 26 educational institutions, and 62 non-faith-based NGOs.

If the estimate of two hundred thousand Americans engaging annually in short-term health volunteer trips overseas is accurate, then the organizations that responded to the survey, with more than twenty thousand volunteers per year, represent about 10 percent of this population. Given the uncertainty of all these numbers, and the difficulty of accessing one of the largest categories of volunteers—members of individual churches who travel sporadically and not as part of a larger organization—it would be impossible to assert that these data accurately represent all short-term international health volunteering from the United States. Yet it is notable that the responding organizations represent a wide range of sizes, with four in ten organizations sending fewer than twenty-five volunteers per year and 18 percent sending more than two hundred. They also follow a variety of different models of volunteer activity and different types of sponsorship, and so describe a substantial portion of a phenomenon that has yet to be fully explored.

Interviews

Either I or my research assistants conducted interviews with 119 people involved in short-term volunteering, including 55 host-country staff members in four countries in Africa, Latin America, and the Caribbean; 15

volunteers; 27 officials of sponsor organizations in the United States; 15 expatriates who worked full-time in host countries and have worked with volunteers; and 7 global health experts.

Interviews with Sending Organizations   The twenty-seven individuals with whom we held formal interviews constituted a convenience sample on the basis of three possible criteria: (1) they had appeared on the list of sending organizations; (2) they had provided their identifying information on the survey; or (3) they were in or near cities that I visited over a few months in 2012—Denver, Miami, Minneapolis, Oakland, and Philadelphia. I contacted all organizations in those cities in advance of my visits and was able to arrange interviews with several in each one. In addition to the four cities mentioned here, where I carried out interviews in person, I also conducted telephone interviews with organizations based in Pittsburgh, Indianapolis, and New York City. Additionally, I conducted in-person interviews with representatives of the two NGOs that accompanied the trips that I took to Haiti and Ecuador, one of which is based in Olathe, Kansas, and the other in Indianapolis. Of the twenty-seven people interviewed, two work for corporations, six for educational institutions, five for faith-based organizations, and fourteen for NGOs. They are thus from diverse areas of the United States and represent a variety of programs.

Interviews with International Staff Members Working Full-Time in Host Countries   In the course of doing this research, I was referred from time to time to "expatriates"—people who have worked or are currently working full-time in host countries for organizations that receive volunteers. This was a good opportunity to gain their perspective as well on the benefits and drawbacks of having short-term volunteers work in their programs. I asked them, usually by e-mail but occasionally by phone or in person, questions similar to the ones I posed to host-community staff members. These expatriates include physicians, country staff for U.S. NGOs or Peace Corps, and community development workers; most are Americans, with a few from France and Latin America. They have generally spent two or more years working in another country—in Nicaragua, Ecuador, Rwanda, Kenya, Haiti, Niger, Peru, Cameroon, and Nepal—and had worked with volunteers arriving in those countries. They were either connected to programs in which I participated (in Ecuador and Haiti) or were referred to me through a process of snowball sampling, in which people I spoke with about the project referred me to those who they knew had been working with volunteers in receiving countries.

Interviews with Experts   In exploring the topic of short-term volunteerism, I was interested in gaining the perspective of individuals who had broad experience in the field of global health or who worked in international organizations such as WHO, Doctors Without Borders, and the International Committee of the Red Cross. Through a series of intermediary contacts, I was able to interview a high-level official in each of these three organizations, as well as several others who had worked in various organizations that formulated policy or coordinated activities in global health (Brookings Institution, Global Health Council, and the Global Corporate Volunteer Council).

Interviews with Volunteers   These individuals were for the most part involved in the same volunteer trips in which I participated, and I chose them primarily because they had had previous volunteer experiences upon which they could reflect and that they could also compare with the current trip. Several were people I met who had recently returned from volunteer experiences. Additionally, I draw on field notes from formal discussions held on each trip among volunteers, in which we reflected on our experiences.

A cautionary note: the descriptions of the practices and philosophies of specific sponsor organizations are based primarily on their own self-reports during a specific point in time. Thus they should not be read as recommendations for or against certain organizations without further investigation, keeping in mind that this is an industry in constant flux and transition. I have used the names of interviewees who work for sponsor organizations or who were identified as global health experts because of their position with international organizations, but only with their permission after they reviewed the quotes attributed to them. If they did not want to be named, I used the quotes but disguised their identity. I have not named host-country staff members because of the greater difficulty in obtaining permission and to avoid any potential repercussions from what they said in confidence.

Appendix B

Recommendations for Having the Best Possible Global Health Volunteer Trip

So you want to go on an international health service trip? The reports of life-transforming experiences are inspiring and the advertisements exciting. But there are hundreds of different options; how do you choose? Let's assume that you want the highest-quality experience, both for your own benefit and for that of the country you will be visiting. And after reading this book, you are even more concerned about how to make that work. What should you consider in selecting a trip? The following recommendations are based on the research for this book.[1]

Before You Go

1. Examine your motives carefully. If your main goal is to travel to an "exotic" location, impress a girlfriend, or party away from home, being a health volunteer may not be for you. International service trips require dedication, hard work for long hours—often in uncomfortable

conditions—and a degree of sobriety! If, on the other hand, your main goal is to change the world, be realistic; your accomplishments during a short-term trip will be limited at best. Have modest expectations and be open to learning as much as you can.

2. Consider your personality and work habits:

    a. Can you work well as part of a team, take orders from a leader you've just met, do what may seem like menial chores, and subordinate your own needs to those of the group and the work requirements?

    b. Do you have the stamina to keep going for long days, particularly in very hot weather and often with minimal facilities?

    c. Are you flexible enough to adapt, once you are in the host country, to conditions and activities you did not expect?

3. Investigate the program as carefully as possible. Look for the following characteristics:

    a. Is the trip you're considering part of a regular program run by an organization that works in the same community on a continuous basis? If this is a once-and-done visit, the value may be very limited, and there is even the possibility for doing harm.

    b. Can you find an opportunity that lasts several weeks? Many host-country staff members I interviewed consider a one-week stay far from ideal, unless you bring specific skills to a context in which they can be put to maximum use in a short time. At least three to four weeks is optimal, since it gives you the time to adjust to the climate, orient yourself to the country and the work situation, and establish a routine for maximum efficiency and effectiveness. You may also have a better opportunity to learn about the country and its people, helping to avoid some of the quick cultural judgments and work errors that can occur in briefer trips.

    c. If it's a onetime surgical mission, are the local facilities adequate for follow-up and treatment of complications that may occur after you leave? If not, reconsider; you don't want people to be worse off because you were there trying to be helpful.

    d. Will you have an opportunity to get to know and learn from people in the local community about the health needs and concerns in their area and how these are being addressed? Mutuality in the relationship between hosts and volunteers is one of the essential characteristics of good service trips identified by the people I interviewed.

e. Are the activities carried out by the program ones that supplement rather than replace local talent? For example, if you're going to spend one to two thousand dollars to do unskilled work, consider sending even a portion of that money to an organization that will hire local residents to do the work. Or travel with an organization that uses some of your fees to hire community members to work with you. And if there are physicians or community health workers who know the community and speak the language, do not compete with them by offering similar services.

f. Make sure that the volunteers who provide medical care are properly licensed at home and approved by the host country (if required). Be very wary of the temptation to do hands-on medical care for which you have no training and which would be illegal back home and unethical in any context.

g. Are the volunteers generally well prepared for and well matched to their activities? An example of a questionable activity is allowing new arrivals to offer health education lessons without knowing anything about the local practices and concerns. Imagine how you would react if a person from outside your own country who had never been there before and did not speak the language came to your community and gave you a lecture on how you should behave! You can *assist* local experts and learn from them; just be sure you're not going to be acting as an expert if you are not one.

h. Does the organization offer an orientation to the country beyond the basics of travel, shots, and what to pack? Does it provide information about history, culture, language, the health needs, and the specifics of the work situation?

i. Does the organization have detailed procedures to ensure as much as possible that your time will be productive and your visit safe?

j. Does the organization do anything to evaluate the impact of volunteers? Ask to see reports on what they have accomplished in the past; testimonials about how wonderful the experience was for other volunteers don't tell you how valuable the trip will be for your hosts.

4. Even if you do not yet have specialized skills or cannot spend weeks away from home, you may still want the experience of traveling to another country to participate in a volunteer project. In this case look for an organization as described in item number 3, and then take advantage of the opportunity to learn as much as you possibly can. Read ahead about the history of the country and try to gain an understanding of what the needs are and why. Definitely learn some key phrases in the local language in the area where you will be working (not just the official national language) and use them whenever you can. It shows you're making an effort and trying to connect, and that will be appreciated.

During Your Stay

This part is easier, especially if you have taken the steps outlined above before you go. The best volunteers, according to the host-country staff members I interviewed, are those who:

*   Work hard
*   Follow the rules
*   Are flexible in adapting to unexpected or challenging conditions
*   Make an effort to understand culture and language
*   Respect the people they work with

Never assume that people in the host community are lacking in skills and knowledge. So much of service assumes the superior capabilities and understanding of the server; this may be based on cultural stereotypes and often results in a less than optimal experience. Host-country staff members cite lack of respect for their training and knowledge as one of the characteristics of the (fortunately rare) volunteers they would rather not work with.

When You Return

1. The ideal volunteer understands the need for humility, both while volunteering and afterward. Specifically, after you return,

a.   Do not claim that you "made a difference," "brought hope to the people of . . . ," or "changed lives," and try not to let your local newspaper, church group, student club, or relatives claim it on your behalf. You may have helped a few people some or a lot (particularly if you have specialized skills and have participated in a program that builds capacity over the long term), or you may have had no lasting impact at all. The frequent glowing reports on volunteering feed into a popular but patronizing narrative that suggests that what poor people need is a quick visit from generous (and often unskilled) outsiders, and that may downplay the local populace's own capacity to solve problems.

b.   Do not claim that you now understand poor people and how different from (or similar to!) you they are or that although they are poor they are much happier and less stressed than the people you know at home. No such generalizations can be accurate about any people, and it's impossible to understand a country and its people after a short visit or probably even after a long one. You are a visitor, a small person in a very big world who is trying to act ethically and do the very best you can within your human limits.

2.   Many volunteers are profoundly moved by their experiences and want to change their own lives as a result. Some people are able to do this, but it is not easy, especially as the experience recedes into the past and the realities of life at home take over. It is helpful to stay connected to others who share your hopes and plans and to find ways to continue to learn about how you can make the world a better place, in your own country as well as in others. There is much that you can do to promote better lives for people in your own community.

If you follow these recommendations, the chances are very good that you will have an excellent experience and possibly make some difference. And have fun as well!

Some other resources that will be helpful and provide greater detail on some of the issues addressed above:

http://www.idealist.org/info/IntlVolunteer/Questions
http://www.ethicalvolunteering.org/index.html
http://globalsl.org/

Notes

Introduction

1. Johns Hopkins University, "Global Civil Society: Dimensions of the Nonprofit Sector," Comparative Nonprofit Sector Project Publications 2, http://ccss.jhu.edu/publications-findings?did=59.

2. Based on Lough, McBride, and Sherraden (2007) and "Independent Sector's Value of Volunteer Time," Independent Sector, https://www.independentsector.org/volunteer_time.

3. Lough (2013).

4. Lasker, Rozier, and Compton (2014).

5. Mohamud (2013).

6. Blackledge (2013).

7. In addition to the survey carried out for this book, I collaborated on a similar national survey sponsored by the Catholic Health Association and distributed to its member hospitals and health systems. Some 89 percent of medical mission organizers who responded to the CHA survey reported that their most recent trip lasted two weeks or less (Lasker, Rozier, and Compton, 2014).

8. Edward O'Neil, "Community Empowerment in Health: Uganda," Omni Med, August 2009, http://www.omnimed.org/clients/omnimed/docs/uganda_omni_med_plan_detailed_v1_8_09%5B1%5D.docx.

9. In this work, I refer to volunteer trips and missions interchangeably as the same phenomenon. The term "mission" is not used exclusively for faith-based trips.

10. Citrin's (2010) work on "health camps" in Nepal addresses the "better than nothing" question.

11. Simpson (2004).

12. Pfeiffer et al. (2008); Foley (2009).
13. Wendland (2012, 111).
14. Boutayeb (2006).
15. Escobar (2011, ix).
16. Butcher and Smith (2010, 31).
17. Smith and Laurie (2011, 547).
18. See Callanan and Thomas (2005).
19. Almond (2012).
20. Devereux (2008); Haski-Leventhal, Meijs, and Hustinx (2009).
21. Caprara, Bridgeland, and Wofford (2007).
22. Griffith (2012).
23. "Manifesto for Volunteering in Europe," European Volunteer Centre, http://www.unv.org/en/news-resources/resources/on-volunteerism/doc/european-volunteer-centre-launches.html.
24. "Global Evaluation," Institute for Volunteering Research, http://www.worldvolunteerweb.org/resources/research-reports/global/doc/iyv-global-evaluation.html.
25. "State of the World's Volunteerism Report 2011: Universal Values for Global Well-Being," UN Volunteers, http://www.unv.org/en/swvr2011.html.
26. Thematic Fact Sheets, UN Volunteers, http://www.unv.org/news-resources/resources/fact-sheets.html.
27. Cohan (2010).
28. Wuthnow (2009).
29. Charles Kenny, "Lies, Damn Lies and Surveys about Foreign Aid," Center for Global Development, http://www.cgdev.org/blog/lies-damn-lies-and-surveys-about-foreign-aid.
30. Nagengast, Briggs, and Misawa (2012).
31. Wall et al. (2006, 559). Obstetric fistula is a severe complication of prolonged labor that affects many women in poor countries and requires specialized surgical experience as well as psycho-social expertise. Wall and colleagues criticize the surgeons who travel to poor countries to operate on women with fistulas but do not have the required experience to do so and may cause further complications.
32. Frenzel, Koens, and Steinbrink (2012).
33. Cole (2012).
34. See Cohen, Küpçü, and Khanna (2008); Burnham (2006).
35. McBride and Daftary (2005); Corbett and Fikkert (2012); Berry (2014).
36. Guttentag (2009, 537).
37. Birrell (2010).
38. Ackerman (2010); Crump and Sugarman (2010).

1. Who Sponsors International Medical Missions?

1. This conclusion is based on my exhaustive but inevitably incomplete Internet search for organizations that sponsor short-term health trips (see Appendix A for details on the method).
2. Jones (2011).
3. These are not specifically studied in this work as a separate entity.
4. Respondents included eighty-nine faith-based organizations (50%), sixty-two NGOs (35%), and twenty-six educational institutions (15%). This is consistent with Lough's (2013) analysis of national survey data in the United States, in which he found that the largest proportion (45%) of people whose volunteer activities were mostly outside the United States served with a religious organization.
5. Bureau of Labor Statistics, "Volunteering in the United States, 2013," United States Department of Labor, http://www.bls.gov/news.release/volun.nr0.htm.

6. Wuthnow (2009, 170).

7. Priest and Howell (2013, 125).

8. Wuthnow (2009).

9. "The Worth of What They Do: The Impact of Short-Term Immersive Jewish Service-Learning on Host Communities," Repair the World, http://werepair.org/wp-content/uploads2013/11repair_btw-_twowtd-_full_report.pdf.

10. IMANA (Islamic Medical Association of North America), http://www.imana.org/members/group-_content_view.asp?group=85705&id=136291.

11. Connolly and Brondo (2010).

12. Centura Health, http://centura.org/About-Us/Mission-and-Values/.

13. "10/40 Window: Do You Need to Be Stirred into Action?," http://home.snu.edu/~hculbert/1040.htm.

14. Medical Missions, www.mmronline.org/our-mission.

15. Steffes and Steffes (2002, 35, 44).

16. Lasker, Rozier, and Compton (2014).

17. Zehner (2013).

18. Rodriguez-Lebron and Rodriguez-Vazquez (2011); Loewenberg (2009); Vaughn (1991).

19. Wuthnow (2009).

20. UIA (Union of International Associations), http://www.uia.org/yearbook.

21. Smith, Ellis, and Brewis (2005).

22. Roberts (2000).

23. Pfeiffer et al. (2008, 2134).

24. See Mort, Weerawardena, and Carnegie (2003); Alvord, Brown, and Letts (2004).

25. "Unite for Sight's History," Unite for Sight, http://www.uniteforsight.org/about-us/history.

26. Heart to Heart International, www.hearttoheart.org/history.

27. Booth (2011).

28. Pfeiffer et al. (2008).

29. Pfeiffer et al. (2008, 2135).

30. Butcher and Smith (2010, 34).

31. Polman (2010).

32. Polman (2010, 50).

33. Carman and Nesbit (2012).

34. Klarreich and Polman (2012).

35. Jones (2011, 532).

36. Thomas (2001).

37. Griffith (2012, 793).

38. Penner (2004); "Renewing America through National Service and Volunteerism," Hearing Before the Committee on Education and Labor, U.S. House of Representatives, 111th Cong. 111–114 (2009), testimony of Richard Stengel, http://www.gpo.gov/fdsys/pkg/CHRG-111hhrg47492/pdf/CHRG-111hhrg47492.pdf.

39. Panosian and Coates (2006); see also Guey-Chi Chen et al. (2011).

40. "Mapping Internationalization on U.S. Campuses," American Council on Education Center for Internationalization and Global Engagement, http://www.acenet.edu/news-room/Documents/MappingInternationalizationonUSCampuses2012.

41. McBride and Mlyn (2011, 1).

42. Dowell and Merrylees (2009, 122).

43. Kerry et al. (2011, 1).

44. Crump and Sugarman (2008).

45. Panosian and Coates (2006).

46. Wallace (2012).

47. Vian, McCoy et al. (2007); "Global Health Fellows," Pfizer, http://www.pfizer.com/responsibility/global_health/global_health_fellows.jsp.

48. "Lilly Launches Global Employee Volunteer Program," Philanthropy News Digest, March 31, 2011, http://www.philanthropynewsdigest.org/news/lilly-launches-global-employee-volunteer-program.

49. Dillon (2012, 107); see also Brønn and Vrioni (2001); Steckel et al. (1999).

2. The Activities and Goals of Sponsoring Organizations

1. Sturchio and Cohen (2012).

2. CURE Niger, https://cure.org/hospitals/niger/.

3. The survey distributed through Catholic Health Association found that eight of the top ten destination countries were in Central America and the Caribbean. Kenya and Peru were the other two (Lasker, Rozier, and Compton 2014, 11).

4. California-based Go Overseas examined Google searches for volunteer opportunities in specific countries and then ranked countries by the average monthly number of searches for "volunteering in (name of country)." The analysis excluded searches within the searcher's own country and most likely does not account for searches that looked for a continent or for a type of activity without specifying a country. There was considerable consistency with the results of my survey; the top ten destinations were India, South Africa, Thailand, Haiti, Australia, the United States, Japan, Costa Rica, Kenya, and Nepal. But it is important to remember as well that these are inquiries rather than actual trips. Katie Boyer, "2012 Official Volunteer Abroad Report," Go Overseas, http://www.gooverseas.com/volunteer-abroad-report. Another study analyzed 698 projects sponsored by 289 different organizations. The projects included came from a Google search of "volunteer projects" and a review of the database of Goabroad.com, an organization based in Colorado, and the results refer to the location of projects advertised, not the number of volunteers who actually visit each country. The top ten destinations that emerged were India, Ecuador, Costa Rica, Ghana, Honduras, Guatemala, China, Kenya, Brazil, and Italy (Callanan and Thomas 2005, 192). Had the latter study postdated Haiti's 2010 earthquake, it seems highly likely that Haiti would have been near the top of their list, as it is mine.

5. GINI Index, World Bank, http://data.worldbank.org/indicator/SI.POV.GINI/; "World Health Statistics 2012: Part III Global Health Indicators," World Health Organization, http://www.who.int/healthinfo/EN_WHS2012_Part3.pdf.

6. Seventy percent of mission organizers responding to the Catholic Health Association survey indicated that they had found their in-country partner through personal connections. An additional 15 percent cited contacts through religious organizations.

7. Timmy Global Health, www.timmyglobalhealth.org/index.php/about2/mission-vision.

8. Alghothani, Alghothani, and Atassi (2012).

9. This is consistent with the findings in Lough's (2012) analysis of the census data; of the volunteers in that survey who spent most or all of their volunteer time overseas, almost half spent two weeks or less.

10. Lasker, Rozier, and Compton (2014, 11).

11. Ibid., 27

12. Muthuri, Matten, and Moon (2009).

13. Alice Baines, "Volunteering Overseas: Don't Get Scammed," *The Travelling Editor* (blog), http://www.thetravellingeditor.com/volunteering-overseas-dont-get-scammed/.

14. Wuthnow (2009, 165); Evert (2005).

15. Campbell et al. (2011); Godkin and Savageau (2003) found an increase in cultural awareness among medical students who had been involved in overseas internships of about six weeks' duration.

16. Hunt and Godard (2013, 714).
17. Berry (2014); Lasker (2015).

3. Becoming a Volunteer

1. Lasker, Rozier, and Compton (2014, 19).
2. In the survey distributed by the Catholic Health Association, results from the same question were quite similar, with the most commonly chosen qualifications being, in order of preference, primary care training, character and personality, medical specialty or surgical training, and cultural sensitivity. In this survey we also asked what qualifications organizers would look for in a future trip. Interestingly, they preferred to have more volunteers with primary care training and somewhat fewer with specialty medical or surgical training or with no specific qualifications at all. Many of the organizers expressed a desire to be more selective in the future than they had been in the past (Lasker, Rozier, and Compton 2014).
3. Ibid., 19.
4. Morsch and Nelson (2006).
5. Callanan and Thomas (2005, 194).
6. "Ghana Program Details," Unite for Sight, http://www.uniteforsight.org/volunteer-abroad/ghana/accra#expenses.
7. Unite for Sight reports that nine thousand volunteers have gone through this training. "Global Impact Corps," Unite for Sight, http://www.uniteforsight.org/volunteer-abroad.

4. What Leads to Volunteering, What Volunteering Leads To

1. Butcher and Smith (2010).
2. See Rodney (1981); Wallerstein (2004).
3. "Global Health Volunteer Program," Foundation for International Medical Relief of Children, http://www.fimrc.org/ghvp/.
4. See Volunteering England, www.volunteering.org.uk/iwanttovolunteer/why-volunteer.
5. Mitka (2006).
6. See, e.g., Wilson (2000); Hustinx et al. (2010); Wilson and Musick (1997); Shye (2010).
7. Clary, Snyder, and Stukas (1996).
8. Rehberg (2005).
9. Colin Rochester, "Making Sense of Volunteering: A Literature Review," The Commission on the Future of Volunteering, http://tna.europarchive.org/20081112122150/http://www.volcomm.org.uk/RN/rdonlyres/6EF238B5-0425-4F99-930E-E7665CAAEEC6/0/Making_sense_of-_volunteering.pdf.
10. Clary et al. (1998).
11. Fletcher and Major (2004); Gage and Thapa (2012).
12. Cnaan and Goldberg-Glen (1991).
13. Stebbins (2009,156).
14. Allison, Okun, and Dutridge (2002).
15. Withers, Browner, and Aghaloo (2013).
16. Lough, McBride, and Sherraden (2009a).
17. Lough, McBride, Sherraden, and Xiang (2014).
18. Sherraden, Lough, and McBride (2008).
19. Musick and Wilson (2003).
20. Withers, Browner, and Aghaloo (2013).
21. Lough, McBride, and Sherraden (2009a, 5).
22. Lough, McBride, Sherraden, and Xiang (2014). Many participants in the early part of the research were not reachable after two years, and comparison study participants who did not go on

the specific programs under study were no different than the volunteers on extent of international awareness if they participated in other international travel experiences.

23. Jones (2005, 13).
24. Ibid., 15.
25. Lough, McBride, and Sherraden (2009a).
26. Ibid.
27. Kraeker and Chandler (2013).
28. Lough, McBride, and Sherraden (2009a).
29. Hudson and Inkson (2006); Thomas (2001).
30. McGehee (2002).
31. Dowell and Merrylees (2009).
32. Sherraden, Lough, and McBride (2008).
33. Elizabeth Niehaus, "The National Survey of Alternative Breaks: Using Both Qualitative and Quantitative Research to Understand Immersive and Global Service-Learning Experiences," September 10, 2012, http://globalsl.org/?s=The+National+survey.
34. Kiely (2004).
35. Lough (2011).
36. "British Gap Year Girl, 18, Teaching in India 'Raped by Two Taxi Drivers,'" Mail Foreign Service, *Daily Mail*, June 19, 2009, http://www.dailymail.co.uk/news/article-1194153/British-girl-18-teaching-India-raped-taxi-drivers.html.
37. Simpson (2004, 682).
38. Ibid., 686.
39. Wallace (2012, 2).
40. Kiely (2004).

5. The Best and the Worst

1. Coulehan (2010, 201).
2. Laleman et al. (2007).
3. Kraeker and Chandler (2013, 484).
4. Lough and Matthew (2013) also found many positive effects of volunteers in their studies with hosts in Kenya and Peru, although the volunteers' average stay was four weeks or more, longer than most volunteer trips.

6. Benefits to Host Communities

1. Martiniuk et al. (2012, 4).
2. Wendland (2012).
3. Ibid., 113.

7. "First, Do No Harm"

1. Hartman, E. (2012, Oct. 15) "For Good or for Ill? Community Impact in Global Service-Learning," http://globalsl.org/for-good-or-for-ill-community-impact-in-global-service-learning.
2. Wendland (2012, 112).
3. Citrin (2010, 39).
4. Green et al. (2009).
5. Wallace (2012, 1).
6. Dowell and Merrylees (2009, 124).

7. Martiniuk et al. (2012).

8. Crump and Sugarman (2008); www.gaspworkinggroup.org, www.forumea.org/ ("Guidelines for Undergraduate Health-Related Programs Abroad").

9. Boutayeb (2006).

10. Farmer (2003).

11. McQueen et al. (2010) surveyed international organizations that provide surgical care in poor countries; 80 percent reported tracking complications and mortality and 89 percent said they had provisions for follow-up but didn't necessarily use them on a routine basis except "as needed." There is no indication which of these organizations are involved in short-term surgical missions rather than year-round programs.

12. Polman (2010).

13. Hollier et al. (2010, 1491).

14. Roberts (2006).

15. Klarreich and Polman (2012).

16. Green et al. (2009).

17. Ibid., 8.

18. Lough (2012) found this very unfortunate pattern among Kenyans who work with volunteers. They were much more likely to consider white volunteers as increasing trust in their organizations compared with black volunteers. See also Perold et al. (2012).

19. Green et al. (2009).

20. Pfeiffer et al. (2008, 2136).

Part IV. Principles for Maximizing the Benefits of Volunteer Health Trips

1. World Health Organization, UNICEF, UNFPA, and The World Bank, "Trends in Maternal Mortality: 1990 to 2010," http://www.who.int/reproductivehealth/publications/monitoring/9789241503631/en/.

2. Farmer et al. (2013, 185).

3. "Comhlamh—Code of Practice for Sending Organisations," International Forum for Volunteering in Development, http://forum-ids.org/2014/05/code-of-practice-for-sending-organisations/.

8. Mutuality and Continuity

1. Nadia De Leon, "Can Critical Global Engagement Be to Colonialism in International Development What Service-Learning Is to Charity in Community Development? Thoughts from IARSLCE 2012," October 10, 2012, http://globalsl.org/2012/10/10/can-critical-global-engagement-be-to-colonialism-in-international-development-what-service-learning-is-to-charity-in-community-development-thoughts-from-iarslce-2012/.

2. D'Arlach, Sanchez, and Feuer (2009, 7).

3. John Saltmarsh, Matthew Hartley, and Patti Clayton," "Democratic Engagement White Paper," NERCHE (New England Resource Center for Higher Education), http://futureof engagement.files.wordpress.com/2009/02/democratic-engagement-white-paper-2_13_09.pdf.

4. Kraeker and Chandler (2013, 485).

5. Wendland (2012).

6. Fifty-four percent said they "always" have a local partner; 18 percent said "usually."

7. Lasker, Rozier, and Compton (2014, 18). The CHA survey found that the most common role of partners is to help with logistics, not to be part of defining goals and activities (p.17).

8. Duenas et al. (2012).

9. Marck et al. (2010).

10. Sykes et al. (2012).

9. Community-Focused Research

1. Welling et al. (2010).

2. Rhodes, Malow, and Jolly (2010); Minkler and Wallerstein (2008); Wallerstein and Duran (2010).

3. Alghothani, Alghothani, and Atassi (2012).

4. Steffes and Steffes (2002).

5. Janet Kerley and Susan Jenkins, "The Impact of Peace Corps Service on Host Communities and Host Country Perceptions of Americans," Peace Corps Office of Strategic Information, Research, and Planning, http://files.peacecorps.gov/multimedia/pdf/opengov/impact_of_PC_service.pdf.

6. For example, Hatry et al. (1996); Sherril B. Gelmon, Barbara A. Holland, and Anu F. Shinnamon, "Health Professions Schools in Service to the Nation: Final Evaluation Report," Community-Campus Partnerships for Health, November 1998, http://depts.washington.edu/ccph/pdf_files/HPSISN%20Final%20Evaluation%20Report&201996-1998.pdf; M. J. Gray et al., "Coupling Service and Learning in Higher Education: The Final Report of the Evaluation of the Learn and Serve America, Higher Education Program," The RAND Corporation, http://www.rand.org/content/dam/rand/pubs/monograph_reports/2009/MR998.pdf; Ferrari and Worrall (2000).

7. Margaret C. Plantz, Martha Taylor Greenway, and Michael Hendricks (2006), "Outcome Measurement: Showing Results in the Nonprofit Sector," Outcome Measurement Resource Network, United Way of America, http://national.unitedway.org/outcomes/library/ndpaper.cfm.

8. "Results-Based Programming, Management and Monitoring (RBM) Approach as Applied at UNESCO," UNESCO, http://unesdoc.unesco.org/images/0017/001775/177568e.pdf.

9. Fortuin and Van Marissing (2009); "Results-Based Programming."

10. Maki et al. (2008) Martiniuk et al. (2012); Sykes et al. (2014).

11. Sykes et al. (2012).

12. The International Forum for Volunteering in Development (http://forum-ids.org/research/) is a source for research on volunteering in relation to development. There are also a few examples of program evaluation tools developed for specific types of international volunteering. Boston University's Center for International Health and Development created the International Corporate Volunteering (ICV) Toolkit to gauge the effect of company volunteer efforts on beneficiary organizations or communities; it was used to evaluate Pfizer's Global Health Fellows Program. The Toolkit comprises a volunteer survey and a partner survey. See Vian, Feeley, McLeod et al. (2007).

13. CSI (Corporate Social Investment) Solutions, http://www.csisolutions.co.za/lbg-model.php.

14. Suchdev et al. (2007).

15. Maki et al. (2008).

16. Alghothani, Alghothani, and Atassi (2012).

17. In the CHA-sponsored survey described earlier, 88 percent of mission organizers reported evaluating the benefit of the trip to volunteers, compared with 60 percent who evaluated benefit to host communities. The most frequent forms of evaluation were informal feedback from host communities and partners.

18. Similar questions were asked on the survey distributed through the Catholic Health Association. When we asked about evidence that might exist of the mission trip's value to host communities where volunteers served, the most commonly selected response was "Partner satisfaction/

invitation to return" (73%), followed by "Anecdotal reports (written or verbal) from partner organization" (66%). Sixty-four percent cited statistical reports of activities, and 56 percent noted appreciation from patients. Lasker, Rozier, and Compton (2014).

10. Programmatic Focus

1. McKinlay (2008. 578).
2. Martiniuk et al. (2012).
3. Hunter and MacDonald (2010); "UN-Water Global Analysis and Assessment of Sanitation and Drinking-Water (GLAAS) 2014 Report: Investing in Water and Sanitation: Increasing Access, Reducing Inequalities," World Health Organization, http://www.who.int/water_sanitation_health/en/.
4. Mbizvo et al. (2013).
5. Austin (2013).
6. Black et al. (2008).
7. Moran (2012).
8. Bezruchka (2000).
9. For example, Rosenberg et al. (2010).
10. Preet (2013); Seymour et al. (2013).
11. Tennant, Kruger, and Jacobs (2010).
12. O'Callaghan (2012).
13. Kiely (2004); Lough (2012).
14. Lough (2012). Eighty-five percent of the Kenyan participants believed that they learned new skills from long-term volunteers, compared with 56 percent who thought that about short-term volunteers.

Conclusion

1. Rafia Zakaria, "The White Tourist's Burden," Aljazeera America, April 21, 2014, http://america.aljazeera.com/opinions/2014/4/volunteer-tourismwhitevoluntouristsafricaaidsorphans.html.
2. Becton Dickinson (2011).
3. Radstone (2005); Ackerman (2010); DeCamp (2011); Dowell and Merrylees (2009).
4. Ackerman (2010).
5. Crump and Sugarman (2010).
6. Vermund et al. (2010).
7. Welling et al. (2010, 467).
8. Nicole Johnston, "What a Waste: Donors Sending Expired Medicine to Gaza," August 21, 2010, http://www.informationclearinghouse.info/article26217.htm; Peter Howitt et al., "Technologies for Global Health," The *Lancet* and Imperial College of London, http://thelancet.com/commissions/technologies-for-global-health.
9. Polman (2010, 55–56). "MONGO" is her term for "My Own NGO."
10. Medical Missions, http://www.medicalmissions.com/network/organizations/jfp.
11. McGehee and Anderies (2008, 20).
12. Heffernan and Fogarty (2010).
13. Abbatuci (1928), cited in Lasker (1977).
14. Caprara, Bridgeland, and Wofford (2007).
15. Butcher and Smith (2010, 33).
16. See Talwalker (2012).
17. Smith and Laurie (2011, 548).

18. Butcher and Smith (2010, 33).

19. Jason Kimelman-Block, Op-Ed: "'Kavannah' Counts in Jewish Service Projects," JTA, January 11, 2010, http://www.jta.org/2010/01/12/news-opinion/opinion/op-ed-kavannah-counts-in-jewish-service-projects.

20. Lough (2012).

21. Farmer (2003).

22. Benatar, Daar, and Singer (2005, 588).

23. Munson (2009).

24. Partners In Health, http://pih.org/youcando/volunteer.html.

25. See Fox (2014).

26. Livermore (2012).

27. Robert Reese, "Short-Term Missions and Dependency," World Mission Associates, http://www.wmausa.org/page.aspx?id=242674; Livermore (2012); Farrell (2013).

28. Lasker, Rozier, and Compton (2014).

29. Corbett and Fikkert (2012).

Appendix B

1. An earlier version of these guidelines appeared on the *Building a Better World* blog, http://globalsl.org/2013/06/03/how-to-have-the-best-possible-global-health-volunteer-trip/.

REFERENCES

Abbatucci, S. 1928. *Médecins Coloniaux*. Paris: Editions Larose.

Ackerman, Lani K. 2010. "The Ethics of Short-Term International Health Electives in Developing Countries." *Annals of Behavioral Science and Medical Education* 16 (2): 40–43.

Alghothani, Nora, Yousef Alghothani, and Bassel Atassi. 2012. "Evaluation of a Short-Term Medical Mission to Syrian Refugee Camps in Turkey." *Avicenna Journal of Medicine* 2 (4): 84–88.

Allison, Lora D., Morris A. Okun, and Kathy S. Dutridge. 2002. "Assessing Volunteer Motives: A Comparison of an Open-Ended Probe and Likert Rating Scales." *Journal of Community and Applied Social Psychology* 12 (4): 243–255.

Almond, Kyle. 2012. "An Awards Show for the Selfless." CNN, November 30. http://edition.cnn.com/2012/09/20/world/cnnheroes-tribute-show.

Alvord, Sarah H., L. David Brown, and Christine W. Letts. 2004. "Social Entrepreneurship and Societal Transformation: An Exploratory Study." *Journal of Applied Behavioral Science* 40 (3): 260–282.

Austin, Kelly F. 2013. "Export Agriculture Is Feeding Malaria: A Cross-National Examination of the Environmental and Social Causes of Malaria Prevalence." *Population and Environment* 35 (2): 133–158.

Becton Dickinson. 2011. *Our Envisioned Future: Assessing the BD Volunteer Service Trip Program, Ghana 2007–2009*, Final Report. Prepared by Corporate Citizenship.

Benatar, Solomon R., Abdallah S. Daar, and Peter A. Singer. 2005. "Global Health Challenges: The Need for an Expanded Discourse on Bioethics." *PLOS Medicine* 2 (7): 588.

Berry, Nicole S. 2014. "Did We Do Good? NGOs, Conflicts of Interest and the Evaluation of Short-Term Medical Missions in Sololá, Guatemala." *Social Science & Medicine* 30:1–8.

Bezruchka, Stephen. 2000. "Medical Tourism as Medical Harm to the Third World: Why? For Whom?" *Wilderness and Environmental Medicine* 11:77–78.

Birrell, Ian. 2010. "Before You Pay to Go Abroad, Think of the Harm You Might Do." *The Guardian*, November 14, http://www.theguardian.com/commentisfree/2010/nov/14/orphans-cambodia-aids-holidays-madonna.

Black, Robert E., Lindsay H. Allen, Zulfigar A. Bhutta, Laura E. Caulfield, Mercedes de Onis, Majid Ezzati, Colin Mathers, and Juan Rivera. 2008. "Maternal and Child Undernutrition: Global and Regional Exposures and Health Consequences." *Lancet* 371 (9608): 243–260.

Blackledge, Sam. 2013. "In Defence of 'Voluntourists.'" *Guardian*, February 25. http://www.guardian.co.uk/world/2013/feb/25/in-defence-of-voluntourism1.

Booth, William. 2011. "NGOs in Haiti Face New Questions about Effectiveness." *Washington Post*, February 1. http://www.washingtonpost.com/wp-dyn/content/article/2011/02/01/AR2011020102030.html.

Boutayeb, Abdesslam. 2006. "The Double Burden of Communicable and Noncommunicable Diseases in Developing Countries." *Transactions of the Royal Society of Tropical Medicine and Hygiene* 100 (3): 191–199.

Brønn, Peggy Simcic, and Albana Belliu Vrioni. 2001. "Corporate Social Responsibility and Cause-Related Marketing: An Overview." *International Journal of Advertising* 20:207–222.

Burnham, Patrick. 2006. "Are These the New Colonialists?" *Guardian*, August 17. http://www.theguardian.com/society/2006/aug/18/internationalaidanddevelopment.education.

Butcher, Jim, and Peter Smith. 2010. "'Making a Difference': Volunteer Tourism and Development." *Tourism Recreation Research* 35 (1): 27–36.

Callanan, Michelle, and Sarah Thomas. 2005. "Volunteer Tourism: Deconstructing Volunteer Activities within a Dynamic Environment." In *Niche Tourism: Contemporary Issues, Trends, and Cases*, edited by Marina Novelli, 183–203. Oxford: Elsevier.

Campbell, Alex, Maura Sullivan, Randy Sherman, and William P. Magee. 2011. "The Medical Mission and Modern Cultural Competency Training." *Journal of the American College of Surgeons* 212 (1): 124–129.

Caprara, David L., Harris Wofford, and John Bridgeland. 2007. "Global Service Fellowships: Building Bridges through American Volunteers." *Brookings Institution Policy Brief Series* 160.

Carman, Joanne G., and Rebecca Nesbit. 2012. "Founding New Nonprofit Organizations: Syndrome or Symptom?" *Nonprofit and Voluntary Sector Quarterly* 42 (3): 603–621.

Citrin, David M. 2010. "The Anatomy of Ephemeral Health Care: 'Health Camps' and Shorter-Term Medical Voluntourism in Remote Nepal." *Studies in Nepali History* 15 (1): 27–72.

Clary, E. G., M. Snyder, R. D. Ridge, J. Copeland, A. A. Stukas, J. Haugen, and P. Meine. 1998. "Understanding and Assessing the Motivations of Volunteers: A Functional Approach." *Journal of Personality and Social Psychology* 74:1516–1530.

Clary, E. G., M. Snyder, and A. A. Stukas. 1996. "Volunteers' Motivations: Findings from a National Survey." *Nonprofit and Voluntary Sector Quarterly* 25:485–505.

Cnaan, Ram A., and Robin S. Goldberg-Glen. 1991. "Measuring Motivation to Volunteer in Human Services." *Journal of Applied Behavioral Science* 27:269–284.

Cohan, Andrew. 2010. "Voluntourism: The Human Side of Sustainable Tourism." *HVS Global Hospitality Services.* http://www.hvs.com/article/4711/voluntourism-the-human-side-of-sustainable-tourism/.

Cohen, Michael A., Maria Figueroa Küpçü, and Parag Khanna. 2008. "The New Colonialists." *Foreign Policy*, June 16. http://www.foreignpolicy.com/articles/2008/06/16/the_new_colonialists.

Cole, Teju. 2012. "The White-Savior Industrial Complex." *Atlantic*, March 21. http://www.theatlantic.com/international/archive/2012/03/the-white-savior-industrial-complex/254843/.

Connolly, Robert P., and Keri V. Brondo. 2010. "Incarnational Theology and the Gospel: Exploring the Mississippi Model of Episcopal Medical Missions to Panama." *NAPA Bulletin* 33:31–49.

Corbett, Steve, and Brian Fikkert. 2012. *When Helping Hurts: How to Alleviate Poverty without Hurting the Poor . . . and Yourself*. Chicago: Moody.

Coulehan, Jack. 2010. "On Humility." *Annals of Internal Medicine* 153:200–201.

Crump, John A., and Jeremy Sugarman. 2008. "Ethical Considerations for Short-Term Experiences by Trainees in Global Health." *JAMA* 300 (12): 1456–1458.

———. 2010. "Global Health Training: Ethics and Best Practice Guidelines for Training Experiences in Global Health." *American Journal of Tropical Medicine and Hygiene* 83 (6): 1178–1182.

D'Arlach, Lucia, Bernadette Sanchez, and Rachel Feuer. 2009. "Voices from the Community: A Case for Reciprocity in Service-Learning." *Michigan Journal of Community Service Learning* 16 (1): 5–16.

DeCamp, Matthew. 2011. "Ethical Review of Global Short-Term Medical Volunteerism." *HEC: HealthCare Ethics Committee Forum* 23:91–103.

Devereux, Peter. 2008. "International Volunteering for Development and Sustainability: Outdated Paternalism or a Radical Response to Globalization?" *Development in Practice* 18 (3): 357–370.

Dillon, Billy. 2012. "Organizational Leadership and the Balanced Scorecard: Lessons to Be Learned from Marketing Activities in a Nonprofit Setting." *International Journal of Business and Social Science* 3 (15): 105–112.

Dowell, Jon, and Neil Merrylees. 2009. "Electives: Isn't It Time for a Change?" *Medical Education* 43:121–126.

Duenas, Vincent J., Edward J. Hahn, Henry E. Aryan, Michael V. Levy, and Rahul Jandial. 2012. "Targeted Neurosurgical Outreach: Five-Year Follow-Up of Operative Skill Transfer and Sustainable Care in Lima, Peru." *Child's Nervous System* 28 (8): 1227–1231.

Escobar, Arturo. 2011. *Encountering Development: The Making and Unmaking of the Third World*. Princeton, NJ: Princeton University Press.

Evert, Jessica. 2005. "Dark Profits? Med School Cash In on Global Health Programs." *The New Physician 54* (6).

Farmer, Paul. 2003. *Pathologies of Power: Health, Human Rights, and the New War on the Poor.* Berkeley: University of California Press.

Farmer, Paul, Arthur Kleinman, Jim Kim, and Matthew Basilico. 2013. *Reimagining Global Health: An Introduction.* Berkeley: University of California Press.

Farrell, B. Hunter. 2013. "From Short-Term Mission to Global Discipleship: A Peruvian Case Study." *Missiology: An International Review* 41 (2): 163–178.

Ferrari, Joseph R., and Laurie Worrall. 2000. "Assessments by Community Agencies: How 'the Other Side' Sees Service-Learning." *Michigan Journal of Community Service Learning* 7:35–40.

Fletcher, Thomas D., and Debra A. Major. 2004. "Medical Students' Motivations to Volunteer: An Examination of the Nature of Gender Differences." *Sex Roles: A Journal of Research* 51 (1–2): 109–114.

Foley, Ellen. 2009. *Your Pocket Is What Cures You: The Politics of Health in Senegal.* New Brunswick, NJ: Rutgers University Press.

Fortuin, Kees and Erik Van Marissing. 2009. "Results-Based Accountability: There Is More to It Than the Right Tools." *Journal of Social Intervention: Theory and Practice* 18 (3): 81–97.

Fox, Renee. 2014. *Doctors Without Borders: Humanitarian Quests, Impossible Dreams of Médecins Sans Frontières.* Baltimore: Johns Hopkins University Press.

Frenzel, Fabian, Ko Koens, and Malte Steinbrink. 2012. *Slum Tourism: Poverty, Power and Ethics.* New York: Routledge.

Gage, Richard L., and Brijesh Thapa. 2012. "Volunteer Motivations and Constraints among College Students: Analysis of the Volunteer Function Inventory and Leisure Constraints Models." *Nonprofit and Voluntary Sector Quarterly* 41 (3): 405–430.

Godkin, Michael A., and Judith A. Savageau. 2003. "The Effect of Medical Students' International Experiences on Attitudes toward Serving Underserved Multicultural Populations." *Family Medicine and Community Health Publications and Presentations* 35 (4): 273–278.

Green, Tyler, Heidi Green, Jean Scandlyn, and Andrew Kestler. 2009. "Perceptions of Short-Term Medical Volunteer Work: A Qualitative Study in Guatemala." *Globalization and Health* 5 (4).

Griffith, James. 2012. "A Decade of Helping: Community Service among Recent High School Graduates Attending College." *Nonprofit and Voluntary Sector Quarterly* 41:786.

Guey-Chi Chen, Peggy, Leslie Ann Curry, Susannah May Bernheim, David Berg, Aysequl Gozu, and Marcella Nunez-Smith. 2011. "Professional Challenges of Non-U.S.-Born International Medical Graduates and Recommendations for Support during Residency Training." *Academic Medicine* 86 (11): 1383–1388.

Guttentag, Daniel A. 2009. "The Possible Negative Impacts of Volunteer Tourism." *International Journal of Tourism Research* 11:537–551.

Hartman, Eric. 2012. "For Good or For Ill? Community Impact in Global Service-Learning." http://globalsl.org/for-good-or-for-ill-community-impact-in-global-service-learning.

Hartman, Eric, and Cassandra Chaire. 2014. "Market Incentives and International Volunteers: The Development and Evaluation of Fair Trade Learning." *Journal of Public Scholarship in Higher Education* 4:31–56.

Haski-Leventhal, D., L. Meijs, and L. Hustinx. 2009. "The Third-Party Model: Enhancing Volunteering through Governments, Corporations and Educational Institutes." *Journal of Social Policy* 39 (1): 139–158.

Hatry, H., T. van Houten, M. C. Plantz, and M. T. Greenway. 1996. "Measuring Program Outcomes: A Practical Approach." Washington, D.C.: United Way of America.

Heffernan, T., and T. Fogarty. 2010. "The Anthropology of Faith and Development: An Introduction." *NAPA Bulletin* 33:1–11.

Hollier, Larry H., Safa E. Sharabi, John C. Koshy, Michael E. Schafer, Judy Young, and Thomas W. Flood. 2010. "Surgical Mission (Not) Impossible—Now What?" *Journal of Craniofacial Surgery* 21 (5): 1488–1492.

Hudson, Sheena, and Kerr Inkson. 2006. "Volunteer Overseas Development Workers: The Hero's Adventure and Personal Transformation." *Career Development International* 11 (4): 304.

Hunt, Matthew R., and Beatrice Godard. 2013. "Beyond Procedural Ethics: Foregrounding Questions of Justice in Global Health Research Ethics Training for Students." *Global Public Health* 8 (6): 713–724.

Hunter, Paul R., Alan M. MacDonald, and Richard C. Carter. 2010. "Water Supply and Health." *PLOS Medicine* 7 (11): e1000361.

Hustinx, Lesley, Femida Handy, Ram A. Cnaan, Jeffrey L. Brudney, Anne Birgitta Pessi, and Naoto Yamauchi. 2010. "Social and Cultural Origins of Motivations to Volunteer." *International Sociology* 25 (3): 349–382.

Jones, Andrew. 2005. "Assessing International Youth Service Programmes in Two Low Income Countries." *Voluntary Action: The Journal of the Institute for Volunteering Research* 7 (2): 87–100.

——. 2011. "Theorising International Youth Volunteering: Training for Global (Corporate) Work?" *Transactions of the Institute of British Geographers* 36 (4): 530–544.

Kerry, Vanessa. B., Thumbi Ndung'u, Rochelle P. Walensky, Patrick T. Lee, V. Frederick I. B. Kayanja, and David Bangsberg. 2011. "Managing the Demand for Global Health Education." *PLOS Medicine* 8 (11): e1001118, 1–6.

Kiely, Richard. 2004. "A Chameleon with a Complex: Searching for Transformation in International Service Learning." *Michigan Journal of Community Service Learning* 10, no. 2 (Spring): 5–20.

Klarreich, Kathie, and Linda Polman. 2012. "The NGO Republic of Haiti: How the International Relief Effort after the 2010 Earthquake Excluded Haitians from Their Own Recovery." *Nation*, October 31. http://www.thenation.com/article/170929/ngo-republic-haiti#.

Kraeker, Christian, and Clare Chandler. 2013. "'We Learn from Them, They Learn from Us': Global Health Experiences and Host Perceptions of Visiting Health Care Professionals." *Academic Medicine* 88 (4): 483–487.

Laleman, Geert, Guy Kegels, Bruno Marchal, Dirk Van der Roost, Isa Bogaert, and Wim Van Damme. 2007. "The Contribution of International Health Volunteers to the Health Workforce in Sub-Saharan Africa." *Human Resources for Health* 5 (19).

Lasker, Judith. 1977. "The Role of Health Services in Colonial Rule: The Case of the Ivory Coast." *Culture, Medicine, and Psychiatry* 1:277–297.

———. 2015. "International Health Volunteering: Understanding Organizational Goals." *Voluntas: International Journal of Voluntary and Nonprofit Organizations.* DOI: 10.1007/s11266-015-9661-4.

Lasker, J., M. Rozier, and B. Compton. 2014. "Short-Term Medical Mission Trips: Phase I. Research Findings—Practices and Perspectives of U.S. Partners." St. Louis: Catholic Health Association of the United States.

Livermore, David A. 2012. *Serving with Eyes Wide Open: Doing Short-Term Missions with Cultural Intelligence.* Grand Rapids, MI: Baker Books.

Lough, Benjamin J. 2011. "International Volunteers' Perceptions of Intercultural Competence." *International Journal of Intercultural Relations* 35:452–464.

———. 2012. "Participatory Research on the Impact of International Volunteerism in Kenya: Provisional Results." International Forum for Volunteering in Development. http://forum-ids.org/2012/10/forum-research-presentation-participatory-research-on-the-impact-of-international-volunteerism-in-kenya/.

———. 2013. "International Volunteering from the United States between 2004 and 2012." Center for Social Development Research Brief 12-08. St. Louis, MO: Washington University, Center for Social Development.

Lough, Benjamin J., and Lenore Matthew. 2013. "Measuring and Conveying the Added Value of International Volunteering." International Forum for Volunteering in Development. Forum Discussion Paper 2013. http://forum-ids.org/2013/12/forum-discussion-paper-2013-measuring-and-conveying-added-value/#exec_summary.

Lough, Benjamin, Amanda Moore McBride, and Margaret Sherrard Sherraden. 2007. "The Estimated Economic Value of a US Volunteer Abroad." Working Paper No. 07–09, Center for Social Development, Washington University, St. Louis, MO.

———. 2009a. "Measuring Volunteer Outcomes: Development of the International Volunteer Impacts Survey." Working Paper No. 09–31, Center for Social Development, Washington University, St. Louis, MO.

———. 2009b. "Perceived Effects of International Volunteering: Reports from Alumni." Research Report No. 09–10, Center for Social Development, Washington University, St. Louis, MO.

Lough, Benjamin J., Amanda Moore McBride, Margaret S. Sherraden, and Xiaoling Xiang. 2014. "The Impact of International Service on the Development of Volunteers' Intercultural Relations." *Social Science Research* 46:48–58.

Loewenberg, Samuel. 2009. "Medical Missionaries Deliver Faith and Health Care in Africa." *Lancet* 373 (9666): 795–796.

Maki, Jesse, Munirih Qualls, Benjamin White, Sharon Kleefield, and Robert Crone. 2008. "Health Impact Assessment and Short-Term Medical Missions: A Methods Study to Evaluate Quality of Care." *BMC Health Services Research* 8 (121): 1–8.

Marck, Roos, Marijn Huijing, Deborah Vest, Mekonen Eshete, Klaas Marck, and Mark McGurk. 2010. "Early Outcome of Facial Reconstructive Surgery Abroad: A Comparative Study." *European Journal of Plastic Surgery* 33:193–197.

Martiniuk, Alexandria L., Mitra Manouchehrian, Joel A. Negin, and Anthony B. Zwi. 2012. "Brain Gains: A Literature Review of Medical Missions to Low and Middle-Income Countries." *BMC Health Services Research* 12 (134): 1–8.

Mbizvo, Michael T., Doris Chou, and Dorothy Shaw. 2013. "Today's Evidence, Tomorrow's Agenda: Implementation of Strategies to Improve Global Reproductive Health." *International Journal of Gynecology and Obstetrics* 121 (1): S3–S8.

McBride, Amanda Moore, and Dolly Daftary. 2005. "International Service: History and Forms, Pitfalls and Potential." CSD Working Paper No. 05-10, Center for Social Development, St. Louis: Washington University.

McBride, Amanda Moore, and Eric Mlyn. 2011. "International Service and Higher Education: Toward a Vision for the Field." CSD Report No. 11–19, Center for Social Development, St. Louis: Washington University.

McBride, Amanda Moore, Benjamin J. Lough, and Margaret Sherrard Sherraden. 2012. "International Service and the Perceived Impacts on Volunteers." *Nonprofit and Voluntary Sector Quarterly* 41 (6): 969–990.

McGehee, Nancy Gard. 2002. "Alternative Tourism and Social Movements." *Annals of Tourism Research* 29 (1): 124–143.

McGehee, Nancy Gard, and Kathleen Andereck. 2008. "Pettin' the Critters: Exploring the Complex Relationship between Volunteers and the Voluntoured." In *Journeys of Discovery in Volunteer Tourism: International Case Study Perspectives*, edited by Kevin D. Lyons and Stephen Wearing, 12–24. Cambridge, MA: CAB International.

McGehee, Nancy Gard, and Kathleen Andereck. 2009. "Volunteer Tourism and the 'Voluntoured': The Case of Tijuana, Mexico." *Journal of Sustainable Tourism* 17 (1): 39–51.

McKinlay, John B. 2008. "A Case for Refocusing Upstream: The Political Economy of Illness." In *The Sociology of Health and Illness*, edited by Peter Conrad. New York: Worth.

McQueen, K. A. Kelly, Joseph A. Hyder, Breena R. Taira Nadine Semer, Frederick M. Burkle, Jr., and Kathleen M. Casey. 2010. "The Provision of Surgical Care by International Organizations in Developing Countries: A Preliminary Report." *World Journal of Surgery* 34:397–402.

Minkler, Meredith, and Nina Wallerstein. 2008. *Community-Based Participatory Research for Health: From Process to Outcomes*. San Francisco: Wiley.

Mitka, Mike 2006. "Volunteering Overseas Gives Physicians a Measure of Adventure and Altruism." *JAMA* 294 (6): 671–672.

Mohamud, Ossob. 2013. "Beware the 'Voluntourists' Doing Good." *Guardian*, February 13. http://www.guardian.co.uk/world/2013/feb/13/beware-voluntourists-doing-good.

Moran, Michael. 2012. "Rethinking Africa's Health, Part I and Part II." *Slate*, May 28–29.

Morsch, Gary, and Dean Nelson. 2006. *The Power of Serving Others: You Can Start Where You Are*. San Francisco: Berrett-Koehler.

Mort, Gillian Sullivan, Jay Weerawardena, and Kashonia Carnegie. 2003. "Social Entrepreneurship: Towards Conceptualization." *International Journal of Nonprofit and Voluntary Sector Marketing* 8 (1): 76–88.

Munson, Ziad. 2009. *The Making of Pro-Life Activists: How Social Movement Mobilization Works*. Chicago: University of Chicago Press.

Musick, Marc A., and John Wilson. 2003. "Volunteering and Depression: The Role of Psychological and Social Resources in Different Age Groups." *Social Science and Medicine* 56:259–269.

Muthuri, Judy N., Dirk Matten, and Jeremy Moon. 2009. "Employee Volunteering and Social Capital: Contributions to Corporate Social Responsibility." *British Journal of Management* 20:75–89.

Nagengast, E., L. Briggs, and B. Misawa. 2012. "Ethical Predicaments of Promoting Student Internships in Africa." Paper presented at Forum on Education Abroad, Denver, CO, March 21–31.

O'Callaghan, Michael G. 2012. "Implementation of an International Short-Term Dental Mission." *General Dentistry* (July/August): 348–352.

Panosian, Claire, and Thomas J. Coates. 2006. "The New Medical 'Missionaries'—Grooming the Next Generation of Global Health Workers." *New England Journal of Medicine* 354 (17): 1771–1773.

Penner, Louis A. 2004. "Volunteerism and Social Problems: Making Things Better or Worse?" *Journal of Social Issues* 60 (3): 645–666.

Perold, Helene, Lauren A. Graham, Eddy Mazembo Mavungu, Karena Cronin, Learnmore Muchemwa, and Benjamin J. Lough. 2012. "The Colonial Legacy of International Voluntary Service." *Community Development Journal* 48 (2): 179–196.

Pfeiffer, James, Wendy Johnson, Meredith Fort, Aaron Shakow, Amy Hagopian, Steve Gloyd, and Kenneth Gimbel-Sherr. 2008. "Strengthening Health Systems in Poor Countries: A Code of Conduct for Nongovernmental Organizations." *American Journal of Public Health* 98 (12): 2134–2140.

Plantz, Margaret C., Martha Taylor Greenway, and Michael Hendricks. 2006. "Outcome Measurement: Showing Results in the Nonprofit Sector," Outcome Measurement Resource Network, United Way of America, http://national.unitedway.org/outcomes/library/ndpaper.cfm.

Polman, Linda. 2010. *The Crisis Caravan: What's Wrong with Humanitarian Aid?* New York: Macmillan.

Preet, Raman. 2013. "Health Professionals for Global Health: Include Dental Personnel Upfront!" *Global Health Action* 6:21398.

Priest, Robert J., and Brian M. Howell. 2013. "Introduction: Theme Issue on Short-Term Missions." *Missiology: An International Review* 41 (2): 124–129.

Radstone, S. J. J. 2005. "Practising on the Poor? Health Care Workers' Beliefs about the Role of Medical Students during Their Elective." *Journal of Medical Ethics* 31:109–10.

Rehberg, Walter. 2005. "Altruistic Individualists: Motivations for International Volunteering among Young Adults in Switzerland." *Voluntas: International Journal of Voluntary and Nonprofit Organizations* 16 (2): 109–122.

Rhodes, Scott D., Robert M. Malow, and Christine Jolly. 2010. "Community-Based Participatory Research (CBPR): A New and Not-So-New Approach to HIV/AIDS Prevention, Care, and Treatment." *AIDS Education and Prevention* 22 (3): 173–183.

Roberts, Adam. 2000. "International NGOs: New Gods Overseas." *The Economist*, 73–74.

Roberts, Maya. 2006. "Duffle Bag Medicine." *JAMA* 295 (13): 1491–1492.

Rodney, Walter. 1981. *How Europe Underdeveloped Africa*. Washington, DC: Howard University Press.

Rodríguez-Lebrón, Andrea Sofía, and Eduardo Rodriquez-Vásquez. 2011. "Las Iglesias Protestantes y Su Obra Médica Social en Puerto Rico: 1898–1930." *El Bisturí* (November): 31–38.

Rosenberg, Mark L., Elisabeth S. Hayes, Margaret H. McIntyre, and Nancy Neill. 2010. *Real Collaboration: What It Takes for Global Health to Succeed*. Berkeley: University of California Press.

Seager, Greg. 2012. *When Healthcare Hurts: An Evidence Based Guide for Best Practices in Global Health Initiatives*. Bloomington: AuthorHouse.

Seymour, Brittany, Ibra Muhumuza, Chris Mumena, Moses Isyagi, Jane Barrow, and Valli Meeks. 2013. "Including Oral Health Training in a Health System Strengthening Program in Rwanda." *Global Health Action* 6:10.3402.

Sherraden, Margaret S., Benjamin Lough, and Amanda Moore McBride. 2008. "Effects of International Volunteering and Service: Individual and Institutional Predictors." *Voluntas* 19:395–421.

Shye, Samuel. 2010. "The Motivations to Volunteer: A Systematic Quality of Life Theory." *Social Indicators Research* 98:183–200.

Simpson, Kate. 2004. "'Doing Development': The Gap Year, Volunteer-Tourists and a Popular Practice of Development." *Journal of International Development* 16 (5): 681–692.

Smith, Justin D., Angela Ellis, and Georgina Brewis. 2005. "Cross-National Volunteering: A Developing Movement?" In *Emerging Areas of Volunteering*, edited by J. L. Brudney, 63–76. Indianapolis: ARNOVA.

Smith, Matt Baillie, and Nina Laurie. 2011. "International Volunteering and Development: Global Citizenship and Neoliberal Professionalism Today." *Transactions of the Institute of British Geographers* 36:545–559.

Stebbins, Robert A. 2009. "Would You Volunteer?" *Society* 46 (2): 155–159.

Steckel, Richard, Robin Simons, Jeffrey Simons, and Norman Tanen. 1999. *Making Money While Making a Difference: How to Profit with a Nonprofit Partner*. Homewood, IL: High Tide Press.

Steffes, Bruce C., and Michelle G. Steffes. 2002. *Handbook for Short Term Medical Missionaries*. Harrisburg, PA: Associations of Baptists for World Evangelism Publishing.

Sturchio, Jeffrey L., and Gary M. Cohen. 2012. "How PEPFAR's Public-Private Partnerships Achieved Ambitious Goals, from Improving Labs to Strengthening Supply Chains." *Health Affairs* 31 (7).

Suchdev, Parminder, Kym Ahrens, Eleanor Click, Lori Macklin, Doris Evangelista, and Elinor Graham. 2007. "A Model for Sustainable Short-Term International Medical Trips." *Ambulatory Pediatrics* 7 (4).

Sykes, Kevin J. 2014. "Short-Term Medical Service Trips: A Systematic Review of the Evidence." *American Journal of Public Health* 104, no. 7 (July): e38–e48.

Sykes, Kevin J., Phong T. Le, Keith A. Sales, and Pamela J. Nicklaus. 2012. "A Seven-Year Review of the Safety of Tonsillectomy during Short-Term Medical Mission Trips." *Otolaryngology— Head and Neck Surgery* 46 (5): 752–756.

Talwalker, Clare. 2012. "What Kind of Global Citizen Is the Student Volunteer?" *Journal of Global Citizenship and Equity Education* 2 (2): 21–40.

Tennant, Marc, Estie Kruger, and Alissa Jacobs. 2010. "Sustaining Oral Health Services in Remote and Indigenous Communities: A Review of Ten Years' Experience in Western Australia." *International Dental Journal* 60:1–6.

Thomas, G. 2001. *Human Traffic: Skills, Employers and International Volunteering*. London: Demos.

Vaughn, Megan. 1991. *Curing Their Ills: Colonial Power and African Illness*. Stanford: Stanford University Press.

Vermund, Sten H., Carolyn M. Audet, Marie H. Martin, and Douglas H. Heimburger. 2010. "Training Programmes in Global Health." *BMJ: British Medical Journal* (Overseas and Retired Doctors Edition) 341 (7785): 1231.

Vian, Taryn, Frank Feeley, William MacLeod, Sarah C. Richards, and Kelly McCoy. 2007. "Measuring the Impact of International Corporate Volunteering: Lessons Learned from the Global Health Fellows Program of Pfizer Corporation." Boston University Center for International Health.

Vian, Taryn, Kelly McCoy, Sarah C. Richards et al. 2007. "Corporate Social Responsibility in Global Health: The Pfizer Global Health Fellows International Volunteering Program." *Human Resources Planning* 30 (1): 30.

Wall, L. Lewis, Steven D. Arrowsmith, Anyetei T. Lassey, and Kwabena Danso. 2006. "Humanitarian Ventures or 'Fistula Tourism'?: The Ethical Perils of Pelvic Surgery in the Developing World." *International Urogynecology Journal* 17 (6): 559–562.

Wallace, Lauren J. 2012. "Does Pre-Medical 'Voluntourism' Improve the Health of Communities Abroad?" *Journal of Global Health Perspectives*, August 1. http://jglobalhealth.org/article/does-pre-medical-voluntourism-improve-the-health-of-communities-abroad-3.

Wallerstein, Immanuel. 2004. *World-Systems Analysis: An Introduction*. Durham, NC: Duke University Press.

Wallerstein, Nina, and Bonnie Duran. 2010. "Community-Based Participatory Research Contributions to Intervention Research: The Intersection of Science and Practice to Improve Health Equity." *American Journal of Public Health* 100:S40–S46.

Welling, David R., James M. Ryan, David G. Burris, and Norman M. Rich. 2010. "Seven Sins of Humanitarian Medicine." *World Journal of Surgery* 34:466–470.

Wendland, Claire. 2012. "Moral Maps and Medical Imaginaries: Clinical Tourism at Malawi's College of Medicine." *American Anthropologist* 114 (1): 108–122.

Wilson, John. 2000. "Volunteering." *Annual Review of Sociology* 26:215–240.

Wilson, John, and Marc A. Musick. 1997. "Who Cares? Toward an Integrated Theory of Volunteer Work." *American Sociological Review* 62:694–714.

Withers, Melissa, Carole H. Browner, and Tara Aghaloo. 2013. "Promoting Volunteerism in Global Health: Lessons from a Medical Mission in Northern Mexico." *Journal of Community Health* 38:374–384.

Wuthnow, Robert. 2009. *Boundless Faith: The Global Outreach of American Churches*. Berkeley: University of California Press.

Zehner, Edwin. 2013. "Short-Term Missions: Some Perspectives from Thailand." *Missiology: An International Review* 41 (2): 130–145.

INDEX